Food As Medicine
The Theory and Practice of Food

by Todd Caldecott
Dip Cl.H., RH(AHG)

www.foodasmedicine.ca

Food As Medicine: The Theory and Practice of Food
By Todd Caldecott

Second Printing – January 2012
ISBN: 978-0-9868935-0-6
Illustrations by Heidi Wilkinson
Photos by Todd Caldecott

Printed in the USA

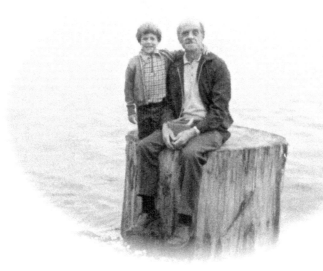

In memory of my grandfather

None of the information in this book is wholly mine. As far as I know I popped into this world as a blank slate, and so I have to thank almost everyone I have ever known that has shared their thoughts on food: from my highschool home economics teacher Judy, my step-grandmother Ethel, my mother-in-law Bev, and not to mention the Chinese shopkeeper on Fraser street that told me how to cook gai lan 20 years ago. But there are a number of people that have had a particularly strong influence on my thinking about food and medicine. These include Michael Tierra, Chanchal Cabrera, Terry Willard, Alan Tillotson and Paul Bergner, and for that I am grateful and humbled. I also want to acknowledge the Nepalese Bajracharya tradition of Ayurveda, including the teachings of the late Vaidya Mana and his son Vaidya Madhu.

As for this present endeavor, it would not have been possible without the loving support and ideas from Lawren Pulse, Neelam Toprani, Paul Kamon, Karen Arbogast, Roswitha Lloyd, Gwen Nagano, Jenn Christenson, Heidi Wilkinson, Alix Rodrigues, Maggie Reagh and Charley Higgins. There are many others besides and in many ways the entire world has conspired to make this possible. But of course I need to thank my incredible wife Bronwen and our three children: Gaelan, Kynan and Kalilah. Their love, patience and commitment to growth and healing provide me with all the hope I need. We should all be as lucky as me. I am truly blessed.

Todd Caldecott
April 19th 2011
Vancouver, B.C.

Disclaimer

Please note that the information provided in this book should not be construed as medical advice. All of the information in this book is provided for educational purposes only, and neither the author, publisher, contributors nor their agents are liable for the unintended consequences of using this information. Please consult your health professional before following any advice in this book.

Table of Contents

4

Section One:
The Theory of Food

What is Food?

It may seem like a rather obvious and simple study, but the nature of food has proven to be a perplexing issue that seems to drive constant debate and controversy. One reason for this is that over the last century society has been led to believe that apart from supplying basic energy food has little bearing on physical and mental health. During this time we have seen farm-fresh whole foods become gradually displaced with manufactured replicas, while bearing witness to previously uncommon diseases such as heart disease and cancer which are now the first and second causes of death (with adverse drug reactions closing in at number three[1]). With the growing realization that human nutrition is a subject far more nuanced and complex than previously appreciated, the reductionist notion of food as nothing more than calories is now in the process of being deconstructed. With this subtlety and complication comes even more questions, and invariably, a lot of confusion.

The centrality and importance of food is resonant in all systems of traditional medicine, including the ancient Indian system of medicine called Ayurveda. In the most venerable and illustrious of medical texts of Ayurveda called the *Charaka samhita* (c. 2nd century BCE), the author recounts the details of a great meeting of medical minds in the Himalayas several thousand years ago. According to this text much of humanity had left off living as nomads and were now gathered in settled groups, engaged in the first attempts at rudimentary agriculture. While this did present several advantages over the nomadic way of hunting and gathering, the *Charaka samhita* states that early human civilization was plagued with chronic disease, and the purpose of this meeting was to understand and debate its cause. Recounting this discussion, the *Charaka samhita* presents each argument of the main proponents, including the notion that disease is caused by individual factors such as the mind and emotions, aging, the environment and genetics. The discussion ends when the venerable Punarvasu Atreya speaks up to comment on the impressive but nonetheless speculative arguments of his colleagues. "It is the wholesome use of food that promotes the health of a person", says Atreya, "and that which is unwholesome is the cause of disease".

While this answer could appear simplistic, Atreya uses it to cut to the heart of the issue. It is not because we identify with illness or are cursed with bad genes that most of us get sick. Nor is it that we become ill if only to bear witness to the compassionate heart of our chosen deity, or by the same token, as the inevitability of our existential plight. Rather, the origin of the vast majority of our health problems is front and center, square in the face, right under our noses and at the tip of our tongues – the very stuff we put inside our bodies every day. Atreya says that rather than invest in speculative theories on health and disease that may or may not be true in the long run, *look for the potential of disease in that which brings about life.*

In the ancient system of medicine called Ayurveda which informs much of my approach to natural healing, the act of eating is seen as a divine sacrament to one's very being, forming and building the structure of the body and mind like devotees building a place of worship and contemplation. Food is something much more powerful than mere nourishment – it forms the essence of your very being. It becomes who you are. You are food.

An Introduction to Ayurveda

Ayurveda is an ancient system of preventative health care and medical treatment that has been practiced in India for thousands of years. The term **Ayurveda** comes from the root words 'ayus', meaning 'life', and 'vedas', which means 'divine knowledge.' Traditional practitioners of Ayurveda believe that it is a divinely inspired practice that teaches us to live in harmony with the natural world by observing and following natural rhythms.

The Concept of Quality

The theoretical basis of Ayurveda rests primarily on the Samkhya darshana, one of the six teachings of the Vedas. It is so ancient that many scholars have suggested that it may predate the Vedic period in India, emanating as an ancient theme that underpins the entire basis of traditional Indian knowledge. The term 'samkhya' means 'to number' or 'enumerate', and in this sense Samkhya delineates the fundamental aspects of reality in a way that can be easily understood.

As part of its structure, Samkhya postulates five elements that underlie all physical reality called earth, water, fire, wind and space. These 'elements' are not chemical elements in the scientific sense of the word, but rather, energetic vibrations that underlie the very fabric of matter. Earth element relates to inertia, water to cohesion, fire to radiance, wind to vibration and space to the absolute pervasiveness of emptiness.

Since the elements relate to function rather than structure, Ayurveda states that they can only be recognized by the qualities they emanate:

- **Earth** is **heavy** and **dry**
- **Water** is **cold** and **wet**
- **Fire** is **hot** and **light**
- **Wind** is **light** and **dry**
- **Space** is **light**

This concept of **quality** is key in Ayurveda, and underpins the relationship between theory and practice. It is through ascertaining the quality of things that we truly come to understand their essence, not in any intrinsic sense, but in the way that one thing relates to another. Nothing is absolutely cold, hot, wet, dry, light or heavy, because all matter contains all the elements and thus all the qualities in varying proportions. According to both the Indian and Chinese schools of philosophy, no thing can ever truly be understood because each contains within it the property of the infinite. Thus rather than trying to base its conclusions on the incomplete knowledge of a thing, Ayurveda is directed to the observation of the relationship between things, and the qualities of interaction.

The following table describes the essential properties and actions of each quality, and the elements that express them:

Quality	Properties	Action	Elements
hot	heating, stimulating, raising	counters cold	fire
cold	cooling, calming, lowering	counters hot	water
wet	moistening, nourishing, filling	counters dry	water
dry	dehydrating, tightening, emptying	counters wet	earth, wind
heavy	condensing, inhibiting, inactivity	counters light	earth
light	expanding, activating, movement	counters heavy	wind, space

The Three Doshas

Ayurveda states that a human is mostly comprised of earth and water, which like mud, forms the grounded earthy structure of the physical body. It is perhaps no coincidence that in many traditions it is said that humans are formed from clay by the hands of the divine. Within this concretion of mud rests the element fire, called **agni**, that mobilizes the natural inertia and heaviness of the body, awakening and stimulating bone, muscle and fat. But as we all know fire cannot burn without air, and so agni depends upon the element of wind or **prana** to fuel the fire, regulating just how quickly or slowly it burns. When the fire and wind elements are in balance the body is filled with vitality or **ojas**, which provides for strength, stamina, energy and resistance to disease.

In a world where nothing changes agni, prana and ojas would exist in a perfect balance, but since we live in a world of constant change they are each subject to alterations in their function. When agni or digestion is disturbed it is called **pitta** (pronounced 'pih-tah'), which manifests as imbalances characterized by hot, wet and light qualities. When prana or neuroregulatory activity is disturbed it is called **vata** (pronounced 'vah-tah'), manifesting as imbalances characterized by dry, cold, and light qualities. When ojas or the innate resistance of the body is disturbed it is called **kapha** (pronounced 'kah-fah'), manifesting as imbalances characterized by heavy, wet and cold qualities. Collectively, these three aspects of physiological dysfunction are called **tridosha**, or the 'three doshas'.

There is a natural tension between the inertia and heaviness of kapha and the fiery pitta aspect that wants to stimulate, awaken and transform the body. The element of wind, regulating how quickly the fire burns, in turn regulates the dynamic interplay between pitta and kapha, like a conductor in an orchestra, or perhaps more simply, like the air-intake on a wood stove. To promote good health Ayurveda states that we want to maintain an optimal balance of all three doshas, and hence, all five elements and their respective qualities. The manifestation of this is good digestion, a happy mind and abundant vitality.

Given the natural cold, heavy and wet qualities of the body the natural tendency is for the fire element to become diminished and weak. In Ayurveda this corresponds to a kapha increase in which heavy, wet, sticky and congesting qualities begin to dominate. Left unchecked this weakness of the fire element impairs the physical process of "cooking" in the body, including digestion and the biotransformation of nutrients. Thus instead of creating physical constituents of the body that promote good health, a kind of toxin is produced, called **ama** (literally 'undigested food') (see p. 212). Figured by Ayurveda to be one of the major components of illness, the presence of ama sets up a predictable cycle of congestion, inflammation, and degeneration in the body. Along with the maintenance of the digestive fire, the elimination of ama through **detoxification** (p. 209) is one of the major therapeutic goals of Ayurveda.

Constitution (Prakriti)

The Sanskrit meaning of the word dosha is 'fault' or 'taint', referring to the body's inherent potential to become unbalanced and diseased. As mediators of the disease process, Ayurveda teaches us that in order to properly prevent and treat disease, we must learn how to identify the doshas and the qualities they manifest. The goal is to restore and maintain the equilibrium of the doshas, and successfully mediate the many effects and influences that can disturb them, such as emotions, diet, stress, and seasonal changes. Although each of us has all three doshas, we are born with a certain proportion of one, two or three of them in different combinations. This unique combination of the doshas is our **constitution**, or **prakriti**.

Kapha constitution
Kapha constitution is more sensitive to qualities such as heaviness, cold, and moistness, and thus measures are taken on a general basis to balance these aspects by emphasizing qualities such as light, hot, and dry. Physically, kapha types have a general tendency to weight gain, with a heavy, thick build. The shoulders are broad and the torso, legs and arms are thick and large; in women the hips are broad and breasts are full. The musculature is well-developed but usually hidden by a layer of fat, hiding any angularities of the skeleton. The feet are large and thick. Facial features are broad and full, and generally well proportioned. The skin is soft and smooth, and the hair is generally smooth, thick and greasy. The orifices (eyes, nose, ears, mouth, rectum, urethra, vagina) are moist and well-lubricated. There is a tendency to lethargy or inactivity, although once motivated the energy released can be very powerful, with great endurance and a steady pace. A kapha type might suffer from a slow and weak digestion *(mandagni)*, as well as minor congestive conditions, such as respiratory and gastrointestinal catarrh. They may display a mild aversion to cold and prefer warmer climates, but if they are physically active they can withstand even very cold weather quite easily.

Pitta constitution
Pitta constitution is more sensitive to qualities such as heat, moistness, and lightness, and thus measures are taken on a

general basis to balance these aspects by emphasizing qualities such as cold, dry and heavy. Physically, pitta types have a strong metabolism, strong digestion, and a general tendency to mild inflammatory states. The body is of average build, with a well-developed musculature and generally less fat than kapha but not skinny like vata. The features are angular: thinner, sharper and longer, with a medium breadth. The skin is often quite ruddy and there is a general tendency to excessive heat. Warm temperatures and hot climates are poorly tolerated. There is a tendency to excessive bile production and gastrointestinal secretions *(tikshnagni)*, loose bowel movements, and more frequent urination. Pitta types are more sensitive to sensory stimuli than kapha, especially light, heat and sound. They tend to be more physically active than the either vata or kapha types, with coordinated, quick and efficient movement, sometimes aggressive, and act with determination and purpose.

Vata constitution

Vata constitution is more sensitive to qualities such as dryness, coldness and lightness, and thus measures are taken on a general basis to balance these aspects by emphasizing qualities such as wet, hot and heavy. Physically, there is a general tendency to being underweight, with dry rough skin, small wiry muscles and irregular proportions. The bony prominences of the skeleton and the veins are easily observed due to a deficiency in the overlying muscular and fat layers. Vata types will usually display a strong aversion to cold, with irregular or poor peripheral circulation. A tendency to more or less constant movement, often confused or peripheral to the situation at hand, including twitching, tapping, bouncing, picking and shaking. The joints often pop and crack, and the muscles have a tendency to go into spasm. Vata is the most sensitive of the constitutional types to sensory stimuli, with poor powers of recuperation and endurance. Digestive powers are typically weak or erratic *(vishamagni)*, with a general tendency to constipation.

Mixed constitution

Constitutional types can also be a combination of two or all three of the doshas, manifesting their respective qualities together:

- **Kapha-pitta** constitutions display a combination of the qualities manifest by kapha and pitta, i.e. wet, heavy and hot. These types generally display a heavy build and a layer of fat seen in a pure kapha type, but they will have a ruddier complexion and more heat than a pure kapha.
- **Vata-kapha** constitutions display a combination of the qualities manifest by vata and kapha, i.e. cold, heavy and dry. These types will often display a lighter build and proportionally longer limbs than a pure kapha, with a greater sensitivity to coldness.
- **Vata-pitta** constitutions display a combination of the qualities manifest by vata and pitta, i.e. light, hot and dry. These types are in many respects similar to a pure vata type, but with a stronger, more compact build and larger muscles.
- **Vata-pitta-kapha** constitutions display a combination of the qualities manifest by all three doshas, i.e. hot, dry and heavy. These types display qualities and attributes of all three doshas, and can be difficult to discern, often displaying contradictory or alternating qualities. Conversely, no quality may be especially prominent, representing an equal balance.

Accurately determining the constitution can be a tricky business, especially when the constitution is a combination of the doshas (see questionnaire, p. 255). Traditionally the constitution was determined shortly after birth and was a complex calculation that analyzed several factors including the ratios of physical proportion. Ayurveda states that because it is the combination of the doshas when you were born, your constitution will never change – it remains a part of who you are for life. But as one lives and accumulates influences there is a cumulative effect upon our body and mind that blankets the native constitution like the layers of an onion, or like a sticky piece of gum rolled in dust. Slowly over the years the body changes and ages, and these factors happen irrespective of our constitution. In Ayurveda this pathological change of the body is called vikriti.

Disease (Vikriti)

While associated with the word 'disease', the term **vikriti** actually means 'change', and in medicine refers to any kind of change in body or mind that is different from normal. In a broader sense, vikriti is the existential fact enunciated by the Buddha thousands of years ago, that no thing, no state of being escapes the winding and twisting road of impermanence and change. Ayurveda is very practical in this way. While it is important to know oneself, we must also be very aware of this cycle of change, realizing that our bodies and the world around us is in a constant state of flux. According to Ayurveda it is this dynamic interplay between life and death that gives rise to illness, disease and suffering.

Kapha, pitta and vata represent the dynamic of change, the ceaseless cycle of birth, life and death that all living beings must undergo. It is a cycle that is replicated on many levels. In the seasons, kapha relates to the emergence of spring after the death of winter, when life is born in the newly green earth, excited by the warm sun that melts the nourishing mountain snow. Pitta relates to summer when the fire element reaches its maximum and the brilliance of the sun calls forth the full blossoming of life, resplendently radiant and powerful. Vata relates to autumn, when the sun begins its slow descent on the horizon towards winter and death, the energy returning to its roots, to the substratum of life, to be called forth again next spring. The daily rhythm reflects this universal cycle as well, with morning relating to kapha, midday to pitta, and vata the late afternoon. In the same way, the first part of the evening corresponds to kapha, midnight with pitta, and vata with early morning before sunrise. Not just the seasons, but our very lives also follow this cycle, with childhood manifesting the softness and sweetness of kapha, pitta the blossoming of full maturity, and vata the slow retreat of aging.

For the practitioner of Ayurveda the cycle of kapha, pitta and vata also relates to discrete elements of physiology and disease. In digestion, kapha relates to the chewing and swallowing food in the upper part of the GI tract, pitta to digestion and assimilation in the stomach and small intestine, and vata to elimination by the large intestine and bladder. In acute illness, kapha represents initial (prodromal) symptoms, pitta the acute manifestation, and vata the chronic illness. In chronic disease, kapha represents the initial stages, as an obstructive, congesting function that impairs normal physiological activities. Pitta represents an immunological response that seeks to restore this balance, inducing the mechanisms of inflammation to remove this obstruction. Vata is the result of chronic inflammation, leading to a loss of tissue integrity, weakness and degeneration. In this way do all things begin, flower and end. Ayurveda exists for the purpose of understanding this, and how best to preserve and protect life.

Like the constitution, disease patterns can also be classified according to tridosha. The specific characteristic of these patterns however is that they refer to pathological, or disease-promoting factors – not constitution. Sometimes the disease is of the same or similar quality as the constitution, but sometimes not. The following provides an overview of the basic disease symptoms associated with each dosha. Combined doshas will display their respective symptoms together, or in an alternating fashion.

Kapha disease symptoms
- Skin feels moist and cool
- Whitish discolorations of the affected area, and/or the face, nail, eyes, urine or stool
- Sweet taste in the mouth
- Symptoms worse with sweet, sour and salty flavors
- Symptoms worse during the beginning stages of digestion, when the food is passing through the mouth, esophagus and stomach
- Congestion and swelling
- Itching sensation
- Dull aching pain
- Pain neither worsens nor improves when pressure is applied to the affected area
- Symptoms worse during the morning or evening
- Symptoms worse with cold and wet weather
- Symptoms worse during spring and winter
- Inertia, laziness, lethargy
- Radial pulse feels wide, deep and rolling; swims like a swan

Pitta disease symptoms

- Skin feels moist and hot
- Yellow, green or red discoloration of the affected area, and/or the face, nails, eyes, mouth, urine or stool
- Bitter flavor in mouth
- Symptoms worse with pungent, sour and salty flavors
- Symptoms worse during the middle stages of digestion, when the food is passing through the lower stomach and small intestine
- Inflammation (redness, heat)
- Burning sensations
- Severe colicky pain
- Pain worsens when pressure is applied to the affected area
- Symptoms worse mid-day and mid-night
- Symptoms worse with hot weather
- Symptoms worse during spring and summer
- Driven, irritable, anger
- Radial pulse feels strong and bounding; jumps like a frog

Vata disease symptoms

- Skin feels dry and cold
- Pale, blue or brownish discoloration of the affected area, and/or the face, nails, eyes, mouth, urine or stool
- Astringent flavor in mouth
- Symptoms worse with bitter, pungent and astringent flavors
- Symptoms worse during the latter stages of digestion, when the food is passing through the large intestine
- Debilitating pain
- Muscle spasm
- Severe colicky pain
- Pain improves when pressure is applied to the affected area
- Symptoms worse early morning and late afternoon
- Symptoms worse with cold or dry weather
- Symptoms worse during autumn and winter
- Exhaustion, anxiety, restlessness
- Radial pulse feels thin and weak; slips like a snake

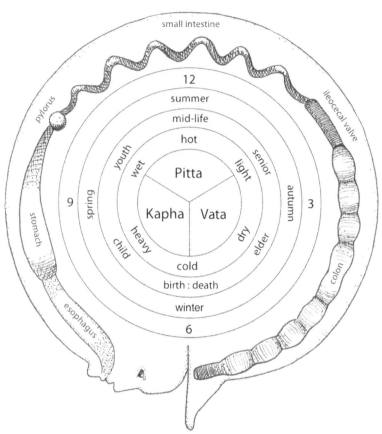

Three doshas in association with the six qualities, lifespan,
seasons, hours of the day, digestive tract and the body

Ayurveda and Food

Along with sleep and sex, Ayurveda states that food is one of the three pillars of life. Most of us know the importance of food, but our consumption patterns are dependent upon many factors besides what we might know about "proper" nutrition. At a base level, most people define themselves in part by what they eat. The act of eating becomes a kind of communion with self, and when shared with others, fosters feelings of trust and companionship. Eating is a kind of truth that we can all admit to, a wondrous fact and necessity of being. Despite this clarity, diet is a highly complex issue, influenced by many factors including season, climate and geography, as well as artificial factors such as culture, urban living and advertising. Our own emotions, other people and external stressors can have a dramatic influence on our food choices. Even the microorganisms that inhabit our bodies could theoretically modulate our nervous system, not unlike like the *Cordyceps* fungus that parasitizes the caterpillar's nervous system. Who is to say that the world of food we have created only serves the purpose of humans? Who is food? Who is eaten?

Given the obvious complexity of food, and the resultant ignorance and confusion that typically follows, most of us end up eating foods that aren't very good for us. Ayurveda is a useful tool that cuts to the heart of the matter, not through the cold calculation of precise mechanisms and measurements, but through a naturalistic approach that actually matches our human experience. The reason why modern nutrition falls short is because it is based upon a model that is alien to the very nature of how we experience food. Clearly we need to have a way to understood food that makes sense and is easy to understand. Ayurveda shows us that through a qualitative approach we gain an excellent awareness of the nature of food, providing us with a set of basic tools we can use to protect and sustain good health.

The Six Flavors

The first experience of food is its flavor, a complex interaction of both taste and smell. In Ayurveda, the basic nature of food is understood through its flavor and quality, which are manifest from six combinations of elemental interaction:

- Earth and water elements give rise to sweet.
- Water and fire elements give rise to sour.
- Earth and fire elements give rise to salt.
- Fire and wind elements give rise to pungent.
- Wind and space elements give rise to bitter.
- Earth and wind elements give rise to astringent.

According to Ayurveda, all six flavors should be found in every meal in order to nourish all the elements of the body, and to maintain the balance of the doshas.

- **Sweet** is cold, heavy and wet in quality, and is found in most nourishing foods, including cereal grains, meats/fish/eggs, milk, fats, sweet vegetables (e.g. root vegetables, squash) and fruits. Sweet flavor balances both pitta and vata, but increases kapha.
- **Sour** is hot, wet and light in quality, and is found in sour fruits and vegetables, as well as fermented foods. Sour balances vata, but can increase both pitta and kapha.
- **Salty** is hot, heavy and wet in quality, and is found in seaweed, fish, sea salt and mineral salts (e.g. pink salt), as well as vegetables such as celery and herbs including nettle and savory. Salty flavor reduces vata, but can increase both pitta and kapha.
- **Bitter** is cold, light and dry in quality, and is found most leafy greens (e.g. kale, endive, chard), bitter melon and in herbs such as turmeric, oregano and dandelion. Bitter flavor reduces both pitta and kapha, but increases vata.
- **Pungent** is hot, light and dry in quality, and is found in pungent vegetables such daikon and radish, as well as spicy herbs such as chili, garlic and ginger. Pungent flavor reduces kapha, but increases both pitta and vata.
- **Astringent** is cold, heavy and dry in quality, and is found in only a few foods such as beans, millet, barley, astringent fruits (e.g. grapes), leafy green vegetables (e.g. chard) and beverages such as tea and coffee. Astringent flavor decreases both pitta and kapha, but increases vata.

[Handwritten margin notes, top to bottom:]
Balances Pitta & Vata
Balances Vata increases Pitta
Reduces Vata Increases Pitta
Reduces Pitta decreases Vata
Increases Vata & Pitta
Decreases Pitta; Increases Vata

Each of the six flavors has a particular effect on digestion:

- **Sweet** flavor stimulates the desire for food, but on its own has little effect upon the digestion, and when consumed in excess promotes heaviness, congestion and mucus.
- **Sour** flavor has a strong effect on digestion, stimulating salivation, acid secretion and intestinal peristalsis. It is beneficial in weak digestion, but is often contraindicated in any kind of gastrointestinal irritation, such as burning mouth or lips, heartburn and ulcer.
- **Salty** flavor stimulates the appetite, promotes the flow of glandular secretions, and assists with the assimilation and absorption of the digested food. Too much salt irritates the digestive tract and promotes mucus congestion.
- **Bitter** flavor stimulates a reflex mechanism on the back of the tongue that results in the synthesis and secretion of bile. Bitter flavor also opens the channels and clears obstruction, but when taken in excess can promote dryness of the digestive tract, as well as send messages to down-regulate or inhibit digestive activity.
- **Pungent** flavor stimulates blood flow to the digestive tract, and has the general effect of stimulating all the glandular secretions, removing obstruction and promoting flow. Taken alone it is contraindicated in any kind of dryness or inflammation of the digestive tract.
- **Astringent** flavor actively inhibits the appetite, drying salivary secretions and promoting the closing of the esophageal sphincter. This is why Ayurveda recommends taking astringent flavored things like tea or coffee at the end rather than beginning of a meal, to block the appetite and stimulate the latter stages of digestion (see p. 79).

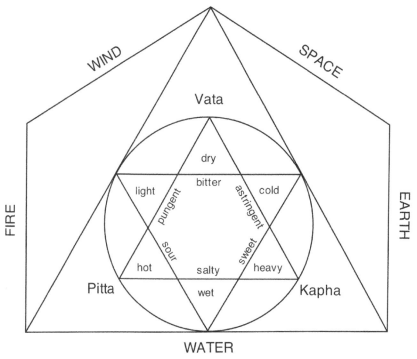

The five elements, tridosha,
six qualities and the six flavors

Season and Climate

The seasons that are created by the changing position of the earth relative to the sun produce demonstrable and predictable changes in the body. While modern medicine doesn't express exactly the same concept, it is well known that certain diseases occur on a seasonal basis. As a result of this effect, Ayurveda states that the diet needs to be modified in each season, and according to different latitudes and climates where more or less sunlight may be present. The sun has a very important influence on our health.

Winter

In winter the cold weather pushes the heat of the body inward, making the digestion strong and enhancing metabolism. Foods and nutrients are thus catabolized much more efficiently and if a proper diet isn't consumed it can aggravate vata. Thus during winter a vata-reducing diet (p. 99) is followed, emphasizing sweet, sour and salty foods such as meat, fish, eggs, dairy, fats, fermented foods and cereal grains. Pitta is balanced in winter, but kapha can be become aggravated due to the cold as well as from the heaviness of the diet. If kapha becomes aggravated pungent flavor can be emphasized in the diet, including spices such as dill, ajwain, garlic, ginger and cayenne.

Spring
In the spring the increasing fire element begins to melt the congested kapha of the body, much like the heat of the sun causes the snow in the mountains to melt. This increase in kapha creates problems such as excess mucus, colds, flu, hay fever, cough and asthma. A kapha-reducing diet (p. 101) is typically followed during spring, eating less fatty and greasy foods, emphasizing lean proteins, cereal grains and legumes, as well as bitter, pungent and astringent flavored vegetables. Vata is generally pacified during the spring season, whereas pitta begins to increase with the sun as it moves progressively higher above the horizon.

Summer
As summer approaches, the warm weather can no longer contain the heat of the body inwards, and thus the digestive fire becomes displaced from the stomach and enters into the periphery of the body, causing symptoms such as heat, burning sensations, fever, irritability and diarrhea. A pitta-reducing diet (p. 100) is typically followed during summer, emphasizing sweet, bitter and astringent flavored foods including fruits, easily digestible cereals, vegetables and soupy legume dishes. Animal foods should be lower in fat, such as lean meats, skimmed milk and buttermilk. Kapha is generally pacified during summer, but vata is aggravated by dryness if the heat is too intense or prolonged. In this case salty flavor is increased in the diet, including vegetables such as celery and seaweed, as well as salted broths, soups and stews.

Autumn
With the approaching cool and wet weather of autumn pitta becomes pacified, but the coldness and the dampness aggravate vata and weaken the digestive system further, promoting the

accumulation of ama (toxins).   Generally a combined vata reducing diet should be followed, emphasizing warming and nourishing foods, predominant in sweet, sour and salty flavors, but along with sufficient bitter and pungent flavors to prevent the accumulation of ama.   Examples include fatty soups, stews, stir-fried green vegetables prepared with salt and herbs, with nourishing whole grains like rice or quinoa, and fermented foods.

Food Quantity and Timing

Ayurveda states that at every meal we should fill our stomach to one half its capacity with food, one-quarter part water, and leave one quarter part empty to allow for stomach churning. In order to do this, the food should be carefully chewed, interspersed with small sips of water, eaten in a quiet environment and with mindfulness so as to become aware of the sensation of satiety. Most of the time we eat too much because we are distracted. We aren't really paying attention to the process of nourishment, bearing witness to the miracle that transforms our food into the body. Instead our focus is externally directed, eating while we do other things, such as working, cleaning, driving, reading books, watching television or using computers. At the same time we are internally besought by emotions that drive us to eat if only to fill an emotional hole, substituting the feeling of having 'enough' for the feeling of being 'stuffed'. Rather than listen to our poor stomachs we listen to the rapacious appetite of the tongue, which in Ayurveda is related to the element of water and quality of desire. The nature of desire is endless, but the body has its limitations. Being able to check in with one's stomach and bypass the noise of the tongue is an important life skill to have.

For the average person, Ayurveda recommends no more than two meals a day, along with a light snack. Ideally, the two main meals should be in the morning after sunrise, and in the afternoon before or around sunset. If desired, a light snack can be had in the middle of the day. This way of eating is better for active people who need to keep their energy going all day long. In some places in India, and also in tropical countries such as Mexico, the largest meal of the day is taken at noon followed by a long rest (or siesta) during the heat of the day. This convenient adaptation is not just to avoid the heat, but helps accommodate the **post-prandial dip** that usually occurs whenever we eat a large meal. Although elegantly suited to hot climates, eating a large meal at lunch doesn't accommodate the reality of the work-a-day world that most of us follow.

Ayurveda indicates that most of our food energy should be consumed by mid-day, when the sun's energy and the body's fire element have reached their peak. Unfortunately most people are in the habit of eating very light or skipping breakfast, grabbing a quick lunch, and then eating all afternoon and evening. The result is that not only do we eat more food than we realize, but we consume it during a time when our metabolism begins to slow down, and thus instead of burning food energy we end up storing it as fat. In my practice I usually find that most people do well by eating a large, low-carb breakfast that doesn't spike the blood sugar, providing a sustained source of energy for most of the day. I find this one simple recommendation to be among the most effective to enhance energy, concentration and productivity in my patients, mirroring the practice of traditional cultures found in cooler, temperate climates.

Food Combinations

Ayurveda maintains a detailed list of foods that should not be combined with other foods. Of these foods one of the most important is milk, which is a complete food in and of itself, and does not combine well with other foods. While it is true that Indian cookery sometimes calls for milk to be mixed with foods, this is not a recommendation from Ayurveda. In particular, milk should never be mixed with fish, meat, radish, garlic, basil, honey and sour-tasting foods. Similar to milk, honey has a number of contraindications in Ayurveda, and should never be mixed with equal parts ghee, with hot drinks and spicy foods. Similar admonitions are also found in China as part of a folkloric tradition rather than a formal teaching. Some of these

Incompatibles in Ayurveda	
milk	fish, meat, radish, garlic, drumstick (Moringa oleifera), basil (tulsi), sour-flavored fruits (e.g. lime/lemon, orange, amla, pomegranate etc), urad (black gram)
meat	honey, sesame, jaggery, urad (black gram), radish, lotus stalk, germinated grains
honey	hot water, ghee (in equal quantity), spicy foods, lotus stalk

incompatible foods include peanut and cucumber, taro and bananas, beef with chestnuts or miso, lamb and cheese, crab with pork or persimmon, rabbit meat with celery or mustard, and honey with onions, garlic, tofu or fish. Although it is difficult to rationalize all these relationships, as a folkloric tradition they are based on real-time observations over thousands of years, and are at least worthy of consideration.

The primary approach to food combining I follow is based upon the chemical properties of the three macronutrient groups, i.e. carbohydrates, proteins and fats, and how they are digested in different parts of the body. **Carbohydrates** such as bread, potatoes and rice undergo preliminary digestion in the mouth with the secretion of salivary amylase, and by mechanical digestion (chewing). They then pass through the stomach unaffected by the secretion of gastric juices, and then on to the small intestine where the secretion of pancreatic enzymes completes carbohydrate digestion. **Proteins** undergo no digestion in the mouth, other than mechanical digestion by chewing, and then pass into the stomach where they are then acted upon by the powerful gastric juices that contain hydrochloric acid and pepsin. The acid and enzymes secreted by the stomach help to break down large chains of proteins into smaller peptide chains. These peptides then undergo further digestion by pancreatic enzymes into amino acids in the small intestine, where they are absorbed across the intestinal wall. **Fats** undergo digestion once they reach the small intestine where bile salts are released by the liver and gall bladder, emulsifying the fats that are then acted upon by pancreatic enzymes. Bacteria in the large intestine ferment non-digestible materials such as cellulose, producing small amounts of nutrients including short-chain fatty acids, biotin, vitamin B12, and vitamin K2 that are absorbed by the colonic mucosa.

When digestion is strong food combinations rarely cause much of an issue, but if digestion is weak, or if poor combinations are eaten continuously, eventually some kind of notable interaction will occur. The biggest problem I see among my patients is the result of combining animal proteins and carbohydrates in the diet, such as meat and potatoes, which require different mediums in order to be properly digested. Enzymes that break down carbohydrates require an alkaline medium, whereas proteins require an acid medium. When carbohydrates are consumed with proteins they inhibit the secretion of stomach acid, or inhibit the ability of the stomach juices to properly act upon the proteins, which are mixed up with carbohydrate. In some people this may delay stomach emptying and prolong intestinal transit time, resulting in the **bacterial fermentation** of the carbohydrates, and the release of gas. This leads to stomach bloating, burping, nausea and heartburn, causing the stomach and esophagus to become distended. If this becomes a chronic event, this distension may eventually cause the outside of the stomach to adhere to other tissues in the abdomen, such as the diaphragm, leading to hiatus hernia. Poor gastric motility and bloating may also compromise the function of the lower esophageal sphincter, allowing stomach juices to rise up into the esophagus, resulting in acid reflux and heartburn.

When carbohydrates impair the process of protein digestion improperly denatured proteins pass into the small intestine. Enzymes released by the pancreas that are designed to break down smaller peptides cannot efficiently break these larger proteins down, inducing bacterial **protein putrefaction.** In the process of digesting improperly denatured proteins, the putrefactive bacteria release toxic metabolites including indole and skatole that damage the intestinal wall, enter into the blood and tax the detoxification systems of the body. Both carbohydrate fermentation in the stomach and protein putrefaction in the intestine place undue stress upon the digestive tract, and set the stage for chronic insult that leads to epithelial damage and intestinal permeability. To avoid this problem, protein and starch combinations should be watched closely. If they are consumed together take them in a way which facilitates better digestion, such as soupy meat dishes taken with boiled whole grains rather than something like a grilled steak and baked potato, or a roast beef sandwich.

Fats also influence the digestion of proteins and carbohydrates by slowing down how quickly the stomach empties. Whenever we eat a fat the body delays stomach emptying so it can begin to synthesize all the bile it will need to properly emulsify the fats. The ideal combination is to eat proteins and fats together, as this delay in stomach emptying helps to ensure proper protein digestion. Mixed with starches however, fat delays carbohydrate digestion, causing it to sit in the stomach longer. For most complex carbohydrates this isn't a problem and it can even be beneficial, slowing how quickly the starchy food gets turned into blood sugar. But when fat is mixed with particularly gluey and starchy foods such as bread, pastries and pasta, the glue-like consistency impairs the activity of bile, leading to poor fat digestion and gall bladder problems.

Poor food combinations also affect the large intestine and the creation of feces. Most people are unaware that upwards of 60% of the volume of a bowel movement are bacteria. Since bacteria are dependent upon whatever substrate is available, changes to what we eat results in different types of microbial ecologies, and hence affects the nature and quality of the bowel movement. Improper protein digestion results in protein putrefaction in the colon, leading to foul-smelling gas and bowel movements. A whitish discoloration or feces that float is indicative of poor fat digestion. Both constipation and diarrhea can be caused by a lack of fiber in the diet, from poor food combinations, and in constipation especially, refined carbohydrates such as flour, pasta and bread.

The Quality and Nature of Food

At one time all food was either wild or grown organically. Of course **organic** food wasn't anything special or more expensive – it was simply a reflection of the relationship the farmer had to the land. Over thousands of years farmers learned to nourish and take care of the soil, knowing that when the land is cared for it yields its abundance year after year. In traditional agriculture the farmer improves soil quality in order to improve yield, but in modern agriculture this naturally conservative outlook has been replaced with the convenience of chemical fertilizers, which not only lack the same diversity of nutrients as traditional composts, but add toxic residues to the soil while leaching out vital nutrients. Grown as a vast monoculture of plants and meat, industrial agriculture is incredibly energy intensive, and requires a chronic supply of herbicides, pesticides and antibiotics just to sustain it. On a global scale industrial farming could be likened to a rapacious tumor spreading across the countryside, synthesizing and releasing toxic substances to kill adjacent cells, conquering vast tracts of land, and sucking up the earth's resources to sustain its ever-expanding growth. It is a strange and dysfunctional approach we have evolved to food, and if we are to survive as a species, it must be changed.

The organic food movement is the first step in this change but unfortunately the extra expense of organic food means that much of it remains out of reach for the average person. Sometimes the issue is simply one of choice. If we can renew our relationship with real food, not just as something to eat but as a reflection of *who we are*, perhaps we might rationalize budgeting a little more for quality food and forgo some of those more expensive conveniences, such as eating out. Of course the most sustainable solution is to grow your own food, whether at home in your garden, on your kitchen counter or balcony, or in a community garden. I envision a future where private backyards and property are replaced by a green common, where neighbors can grow food together, learning from and sharing with other. Ultimately the solution to the food crisis that faces us will come from simple local solutions, and a new awareness of the inextricable bond between food, life and each other.

The following is a compendium of the basic food groups, including water, fruit, vegetables, meat, dairy, cereal grains, legumes, nuts and seeds, fats and sweeteners, as well as tea, chocolate, coffee and alcohol.

Water

Water has long been recognized in traditional medicine as the source of life, and without it we would scarcely survive for more than a few days. Every system of traditional medicine paid great respect to water, for its importance and restorative effects, as well as its different attributes depending on its source and further processing. Ever since the dawn of human civilization the protection and maintenance of clean, uncontaminated water sources has always been the first priority. In India we can see evidence of this in archeological remains of Harrapa and Moenjodharo, which had a water distribution and sewage network as early as 5000 years ago. Where culture is advanced and evolved, water quality is considered a human right – and where industry and profit supersede this concern the society begins to self-destruct. In many respects, ensuring clean drinking water is the highest expression of human culture.

In the natural world water comes in many forms, and among these types Ayurveda considers freshly collected **rainwater** to be among the best sources. According to Ayurveda fresh rainwater is said to be rejuvenating, strength-promoting, life-giving, contentment-inducing, intellect-enhancing and balancing to all three doshas. If you have never tasted freshly collected rainwater it is quite remarkable indeed. The fresh rainwater collected during a thunderstorm in particular has an effervescent and fertile quality: slightly earthy but more ethereal and dynamic than terrestrial water. In modern times however, rain often contains the residue of airborne industrial pollutants and may not be safe. Since weather patterns vary greatly and industrial pollutants are dispersed across the entire surface of the earth, just because one may live in a pristine environment does not mean that the rainwater is not contaminated.

According to Ayurveda **glacial water** from fast-flowing rivers is considered to be the best substitute for rainwater. It is said to be rejuvenating and balancing to all three doshas. Considering that the water from melting glaciers is of ancient origin, it is among the most pure sources of water on earth. Melting from pristine glaciers, glacial water crashes down steep slopes as a storm of negative ions, filled with the mineral-rich silt or 'milk' of the abraded rock bed. Many traditional cultures including the famed Hunzakuts of the Hunza valley use this glacial milk as both a food supplement and to enhance soil nutrition. I spent several weeks in Hunza in 1990 recovering from a severe case of chronic dysentery I acquired in India. Every day I would walk down to the river to drink several liters of water, and eat the local bread, soups and stews prepared with glacial milk. Within a week I felt re-invigorated and nourished, and could literally feel new life flowing into my limbs. Like Ayurveda I believe that glacial water is a dynamically alive and highly nutritive substance. Many of the longest-lived and healthiest peoples reside high up in the mountains next to glaciers, including the traditional peoples of the Andes, Alps, Caucasus and Himalayan ranges. While they can be challenging places to live, these areas contain the raw vitality and power of the earth in all its abundance, and this quality is reflected in the water.

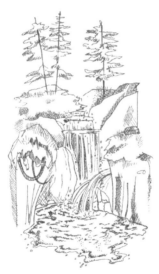

Another exceptional water source are **artesian wells** that tap equally ancient sources of water, in some cases several thousand or even millions of years old. Stored in confined aquifers of rock such as limestone and sandstone, artesian well water is often a rich source of soluble minerals, and like glacial water, its regular consumption is similarly associated with enhanced longevity.

Unlike unconfined aquifers that recharge relatively quickly from surface water, artesian aquifers recharge very slowly and are susceptible to over-exploitation.

While glacial water and artesian wells are the best sources of water, most people in the world rely on run-off from melting snow and the **surface water** that is collected in unconfined aquifers, streams, rivers and lakes. Although these can be acceptable sources, there is a much greater risk for contamination from sewage as well as agricultural or industrial pollutants. According to a recent analysis of drinking water quality by the *New York Times*, the water delivered to more than 49 million people in the United States contains unacceptably high concentrations of toxins including arsenic, tetrachloroethylene and uranium, with precious little enforcement of water quality standards.[2] Even in cities where the water quality is generally pretty good there is always some degree of contamination, such as from silt and dirt during the rainy months, naturally occurring bacteria that build up on the sides of pipes, as well as the chlorine that is added to disinfect the water. Where water quality cannot be assured my general recommendation is to use some kind of carbon-filter (NSF/ANSI Standard 53) for municipal sources of water to at least remove the chlorine. **Chlorine** is well established as a highly reactive oxidizing compound in chemistry, and its purpose in our drinking water is to make it abiotic, or incapable of supporting life, which raises a few questions when it comes to our own health. Apart from the inherent risk of chlorine itself when used in the preparation of food and beverages, it results in the formation of trihalomethanes (THMs), a class of chemical compounds directly linked to infertility and cancer.[3] It shouldn't be too much of a stretch to see that chlorine poses some risks to health, and should not be consumed regularly. Ideally all water piped into your home, including the water you bathe and shower in, should be filtered to remove the chlorine.

Simple carbon filtration however may not be enough in regions where the water is overtly contaminated. In many municipalities **fluoride** is added to the water for its purported benefits to dental health, but there is enough divergence of opinion to question this claim, with activists linking fluoride consumption to many diseases including brain damage, thyroid dysfunction and cancer.[4] To properly remove all industrial chemicals including fluoride either a **reverse osmosis membrane** (with a carbon pre-filter) or **distillation** is required. In both cases however, this rather severe process of purification removes dissolved minerals in the water, turning it into a highly active solvent. Consuming this kind of water regularly will rob your body of minerals, but you can ameliorate this by either using it to make mineral rich broths (e.g. bones, seaweed) and herbal teas (e.g. nettle), or by fortifying it with ionic trace-minerals. I also give this same advice to people living in regions where the water is acidic and soft, or receive their water from desalination plants, to neutralize the acidic pH.

Water purity has been a pressing concern in India for thousands of years, and through Ayurveda certain practices developed thousands of years ago are still used to maintain water quality. For example many people in India store their water in copper vessels overnight, believing that **copper** has a special ability to purify negative energies. Modern research has verified this belief, demonstrating that enough copper ions are released into the water to elicit a measurable and yet safe antibacterial activity.[5] Likewise Ayurveda states that when water is exposed to the rays of the sun all day, and then exposed to the light of the moon all night, it has a special healing property. Research on **solar water disinfection (SODIS)** supports this practice, harnessing the antibacterial properties of ultraviolet and infrared radiation by filling clear glass bottles with water, and then letting them sit in the hot sun for at least six hours.[6]

Ayurveda states that when water is consumed in excessive amounts it tends to weaken digestion, and thus the injunction of consuming eight glasses of water a day is not necessarily appropriate for every person in every circumstance. The best guide to water consumption is to rely on your desire for it (e.g. thirst), and to watch for symptoms associated with dehydration such as dryness of the oral cavity, constipation, headache, or low blood pressure. Consuming water before eating inhibits digestive function and promotes weight loss, whereas consuming water after meals is stated to promote congestion and weight gain. Ayurveda recommends drinking small amounts of water with meals to enhance digestive function and balance metabolism. Consuming large amounts of water on an empty stomach has diuretic and mildly laxative properties, and is a good thing to do first thing in the morning, with a little lemon juice, cayenne pepper or triphala to augment its cleansing benefits (see p. 215). Generally speaking, the need for water increases with bodily and environmental heat, such as with fever or in summer, and decreases with physical coldness and during winter.

Cold water is best to relieve the effects of heat and poison, and is useful for intoxication, exhaustion, fainting, fatigue, vertigo, thirst, heat, and sunstroke. Cold water however is contraindicated in constipation, flatulence, throat diseases, fevers, rhinitis, upper respiratory tract infections, coughs, hiccough, chest pain, urinary tract disorders, cataracts, anorexia, anemia, poor circulation, and tumors. Ayurveda states that cold water should be avoided when eating any fatty food, as it turns the fat into a kind of poison (ama) that the body can't digest.

Warm water stimulates digestive function, soothes throat irritation, cleanses the urinary tract, relieves hiccough and dispels intestinal fermentation, gas and bloating. Hot water is particularly useful in colds, flu and fever, but is contraindicated in physical and mental exhaustion, convulsions, bronchial asthma, hunger, and hemorrhage.

Vegetables

The foundational triad upon which modern nutrition rests is the separation of food into three basic components called carbohydrates, proteins and fats. These are known as the macronutrients, the articles in our diet that supply us with food energy or 'calories', as opposed to the other category of micronutrients that do not. Although not specifically implied, this unfortunate division has led people to think that the macronutrients are more important, more vital to get through the day, giving us the energy we need to get things done. But based on my experience with patients, my feeling is that this tripod upon which modern nutrition rests is a little shaky, and doesn't fully account for what people really need to know about their diet. What I tell my patients is that along side carbohydrates, proteins and fats there is a fourth leg to this equation, forming a solid earthy square upon which our concept of nutrition can be solidly built. Yes it is true that this food may not give you much energy, but as I aim to illustrate, it does have a number of vitally important functions. It is the very food that your mother harped on at you about eating. In Latin it is derived from the word 'vegere', which literally means 'to live', and so I know it is more than just my bias when I say that the most important foods are your vegetables.

Although most of us are familiar with a few different types of vegetables (for some, as instruments of torture), the word 'vegetable' in fact relates to the entire plant kingdom, a surprisingly large number of which are completely edible. Where I live in the Pacific Northwest the local Salishan peoples chose from hundreds of different local plants as food, including roots and tubers like springbank clover *(Trifolium wormskjoldii)* and kamchatka lily *(Fritillaria camschatcensis)*, the young green shoots of salmonberry *(Rubus spectabilis)* and fireweed *(Epilobium angustifolium)*, the inner bark of western hemlock *(Tsuga canadensis)*, and a variety of different seaweeds and lichens. But when I look at what most of us conventionally call 'vegetables', such as the ones found in your local grocery store, the diversity is very limited in comparison, usually only those that have been bred to survive the infrastructure of industrial agriculture such as peas, potatoes and carrots.

As we probe the subject of vegetation one thing that should be dispelled at the outset is this confusion between a fruit and a vegetable. A fruit is the reproductive part of a plant, whereas a vegetable is the part of the plant that 'vegetates', or grows. There is no essential difference between them, except in what part of the plant they come from, and hence, a zucchini or green bean is as much a fruit as is an apple or mango. What public policy experts have done by admonishing us to eat plenty of "fruits and vegetables" is create a mindset that says that the very sweetest spectrum of vegetation should be given equal if not leading preference to the huge diversity of non-sweet vegetation that we could choose instead. Given that many of the fruits we eat nowadays have been selectively hybridized for traits such as sweetness and a lack of fiber (e.g. bananas, seedless grapes), this unfortunate policy essentially advocates for increased sugar intake through excess fruit consumption, contributing to the epidemic of obesity and diabetes that now affects the entire world. What the dietary experts should have told us was to eat plenty of vegetation in all shapes, sizes and colors, but only a little bit of the sweet ones.

In my practice I make a general separation between what I call starchy and non-starchy vegetables. **Starchy vegetables** include potato, taro/dasheen, sweet potato, yam, cassava, carrot, beet and onion, all of which are rich in carbohydrates. For the plant, the starch in a root or tuber serves a vitally important function, allowing it to store the energy it has gathered through photosynthesis – but there are naturally 'wild' limitations on this. Just as we have done with the sweet fruits, we have cleverly found a way to bypass these natural limits through genetic selection and hybridization, dramatically increasing traits such as starchiness. For example, the pinky-orange flesh of the modern carrot bears little resemblance to the ancestral carrot, *Daucus carota*, which produces a small bitter tasting root with rather more medicinal than food-like properties. And yet as bizarre as it may seem, very few of the roots and tubers we eat nowadays bear any resemblance to their wild predecessors, which our ancestors began to cultivate a few thousand years ago. Not that this is necessarily a bad thing, but it is something to be aware of. In preference to eating only very starchy roots and tubers such as the potato, and especially in folks trying to maintain a healthy blood sugar, I emphasize colorful, fiber-rich, lower-starch options including burdock, beets, turnips, rutabaga, daikon, radish, sweet potato, onion, garlic, ginger and turmeric. Fortified with a diverse array of immune-boosting nutrients these roots and tubers, as well as their peels, contain an abundance of fiber that not only slows down the absorption of carbohydrates to regular blood sugar, but also helps to establish and maintain a healthy bacterial ecology in the gut, alleviating problems such as constipation.

Non-starchy vegetables are those which contain relatively little starch and are typically rich in an abundant array of vitamins and minerals, as well as phytonutrients, a class of compounds in plants that have a diverse array of functions in your body, everything from regulating metabolism and preventing cancer, to stabilizing blood sugar and dispelling inflammation. If we can for a moment contemplate the unity of all living things, it is easy to see that just as the flower of a plant corresponds to our sexual organs, the vegetative part of a plant is biologically analogous to our own bodies. Fresh vegetables represent the very essence of living energy on earth, and unlike dried nuts, seeds, grains and meat, are closest to life itself, to the soil of creation and the memory of growth and living. Eating fresh vegetables isn't just good for you, it is a crucial reminder to your body of how to live in the full expression of life. Like roots and tubers, non-starchy vegetables should ideally be as diverse as possible, expressing a rainbow of colors, each of which represents a distinct class of phytonutrients with uniquely beneficial properties.

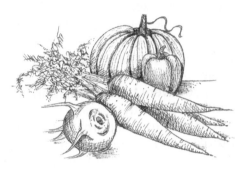

My most common recommendations for vegetables include:

- leafy greens: cabbage, chard, kale, rapini, sui choy, yu choy, bok choy, gai lan, amaranth greens, spinach, lettuce, radicchio, watercress, dandelion greens, beet greens, nettle
- flowers: broccoli, artichoke, brussel sprout, cauliflower, tiger lily, nasturtium
- stems: celery, asparagus, leek, rhubarb, fiddlehead
- fruits: cucumber, eggplant, bell pepper, squash, gourds, tomato, avocado
- roots: beet root, rutabaga, daikon, carrot, Jerusalem artichoke, burdock, parsnip, radish, ginger, onion, garlic, shallot, sweet potato, water chestnut, lotus
- seaweed: nori, wakame, hijiki, kombu, dulse, kelp, bladderwrack
- sprouts: broccoli sprouts, onion sprouts, garlic sprouts, alfalfa sprouts, red clover sprouts, mung sprouts
- culinary herbs: basil, oregano, marjoram, thyme, rosemary, cilantro, mint, bay leaves, curry leaf, fenugreek (methi)

Among all the different foods, vegetables are the most closely allied with medicinal plants. Some vegetables such as ginger and garlic straddle the definition between food and medicine, and can also be used to treat disease. Garlic for example has potent antimicrobial properties, and has been shown to normalize blood lipids in vascular disease. Similarly, ginger has been shown to effectively treat nausea as well as reduce inflammation. Medicinal benefits can be found in almost all plants – the only determining factor is dosage. Plants like basil, garlic and ginger exert their benefits at relatively small doses, whereas vegetables such as broccoli or kale need to be consumed in liberal amounts to receive their benefits. As a general rule of thumb, I encourage all my patients to eat lots of vegetables; ideally, one half the volume of food they eat each day. This means if you were to look at a dinner plate, at least half your plate would be filled with veggies. The net benefit of eating this way not only relates to an optimal intake of a broad array of healthful, antioxidant compounds, but because of all the plant fiber, leads to the satiation of appetite without consuming excess calories.

Although all vegetables are generally beneficial, Ayurveda attributes different properties to each, and hence each type of vegetable has a unique property that can affect the body in different ways. Overall, most vegetables are cooling to the body, which is why they generally need to be cooked a little, to 'warm' them up, especially if the digestion is weak. A few vegetables such as garlic or onions are warming or pungent in nature, and especially in people that suffer from excess heat or burning sensations, either need to be avoided or processed by cooking to sublimate their properties. The following provides an overview of which vegetables can be used to balance the doshas in Ayurveda:

- **Kapha** is balanced by emphasizing non-starchy vegetables such as leafy greens prepared without fat, steamed or in soups, adding in pungent, warming and stimulating herbs such as basil, oregano and ginger. Sweet and starchy vegetables should be limited.
- **Pitta** is balanced by giving preference to non-starchy vegetables prepared raw, juiced or lightly steamed, along with some starchy sweet vegetables like sweet potato and squash. Pungent vegetables such as garlic, mustard greens, bell peppers and tomatoes should be limited.

- **Vata** is balanced by eating more sweet vegetables such as roots and tubers, lightly stir-frying greens and non-starchy veggies in a little fat like ghee or olive oil, along with digestive herbs, e.g. cumin, black mustard seed, garlic, basil, oregano, ginger, salt, wine, tamari, etc. Raw vegetables, as well as vegetables prepared without moisture (i.e. baked or grilled) should be limited.

Please refer to Appendix III: Vegetables (p. 259) for a complete listing of their qualities, flavors and effects upon the doshas.

Fruit

Fruit is something quite special. Although it has a precise and decidedly neutral meaning in botanical terms, the word connotes something much more sensuous, tasty and sweet. It is symbolic of the full expression of life, so pregnant and juicy, so full of possibility and nourishment. This vision of fruit finds its way into our collective mythos as a symbol of sexuality as well as misadventure, such as Persephone and the pomegranate, or Eve and the apple. From a dietary perspective the duality posited by these tales suggests the true nature of what we call fruit, and how we should respect it.

In general fruits tend to have a sweet flavor and cool quality, and help to reduce excess heat and dryness. It is no accident that most fruits are generally produced during the warm season and in warm climates when pitta and vata are increased. The cooling quality of fruit can make it difficult to digest, and thus measures can be taken to balance this property, such as eating fruit with different herbs and spices (p. 198). Outside of summer or a hot climate Ayurveda does not recommend eating much fruit as its cool quality serves to remind the body to slow down metabolism. Rather than eat raw fruit at these times Ayurveda recommends dried fruit, but only after it has been boiled or stewed, which is a useful way to balance vata and nourish the blood (p. 199). Uncooked dried fruit should be avoided due to the difficulty it presents to digestion, as well as the unavoidable presence of yeasts and molds on the fruit that can disrupt the gut ecology.

While fruit has always been an important part of the human diet, it is important to note just how radically fruit has changed. Over the last several thousand years, and especially in the last 100 years, humans have actively bred out characteristics in fruit that balance their sugar content, such as peel thickness, fruit pulpiness and seed content. The modern banana for example is quite unlike its ancestor, which is nowhere near as sweet and big, and contains large seeds that make it almost inedible. Similarly, the modern apple and especially super-sweet hybrids like Ambrosia or Gala are quite unlike their crab-apple ancestors, which are bitter and sour in flavor, and have thick skins and big seeds. The reality is that most of the fruit we eat nowadays isn't really so different than a feedlot cow; bloated and bursting with sugar, but lacking real nutrition.

The best relationship to have with fruit is a moderate one; consuming it in relatively small amounts, and mostly in the summer when it's locally available and your body craves need that cooling, wet quality. Of course not all fruits have this activity, such as sour fruits, which tend to have a more balanced action between cooling and stimulating. In my practice I tend to recommend what I call **half-sweet fruits** that naturally have less sugar, and limit very sweet fruits such as mango, banana, sweet oranges, papaya, dates and pineapple. Following this directive, the best fruits for occasional consumption include:

- wild fruits: crabapple, saskatoon, huckleberry, elderberry, juneberry, Oregon grape, hawthorn, Indian plum, salal
- cultivated berries: raspberry, strawberry, cranberry, blueberry, currant
- pomes: apple, pear, quince
- stone fruits: apricot, peach, plum, cherry
- grape (not seedless)
- melons: cantaloupe, honeydew
- citrus: lime, lemon, grapefruit
- tropical fruits: passionfruit, guava, starfruit, açaí, dragonfruit, mangosteen, pomegranate, prickly pear
- stewed dried fruit: goji, amla, raisin, fig, prune, mulberry

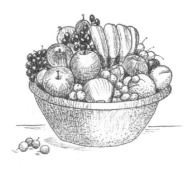

In Ayurveda, most fruits generally balance pitta and increase kapha and vata. Sour fruits such as lemon, lime or grapefruit tend to balance kapha or vata to the same degree, and due to the heat-generating properties of the sour flavor, tend to aggravate pitta. As previously stated, raw fruit is generally too cooling to balance vata and is best prepared by baking or stewing (p. 199) or otherwise preparing with herbs and spices to make a fruit chat (p. 198).

Please refer to Appendix IV: Fruit (p. 261) for a complete listing of their qualities, flavors and effects upon the doshas.

Meat

If any food could be said to define the evolution of the human species it must surely be meat. When we consider our origin as tree-dwelling primates that gradually moved onto the African savanna, the only logical way by which we could have supported the rapid development of our comparatively large brains was to have a local abundance of high quality nutrition, rich in proteins and fats. Apart from the fact that our closest primate relatives including bonobos and chimpanzees eat meat, the archeological record clearly demonstrates meat-eating among early humans, moving up the food chain from insects, reptiles and rodents, to hunting much larger animals such as deer and even the mighty mammoth. Eating meat is not only a native part of our diet, but when considering the social organization required for hunting or fishing, it underpins the very basis of human collectivism that makes us unique among primates.

Meat is lauded as the prime source of nutrition in every system of traditional medicine, with systems like Tibetan and

Chinese medicine supplying a meticulously detailed exegesis of the different classifications of animal products, based on source or part. Even in the supposedly vegetarian Ayurveda, the ancient texts are replete with references to meat eating, and every disease described in Ayurveda mentions the utility of some kind of meat product in its treatment. Meat and animal products are the most tissue-nourishing and anabolic of all the foods, promoting heaviness, greasiness and warmth of body. In all the Eastern systems of medicine, including Unani and ancient Egyptian medicine, meat and animal products are considered to nourish the vital essence. It is the medicine of choice in any kind of deficiency, with the specific types recommended on the basis of factors such as climate, geography, disease or constitution.

In a world where government policy is to have the population eat grains and cereals as their primary source of nutrition (i.e. forming the bottom of the 'food pyramid'), which includes by extension all the refined cereals and carbohydrate-rich products that keeps the food industry in business, meat and animal products have become a convenient scapegoat. Epidemiological studies that purport to draw a link between **red meat** and diseases like cancer and heart disease fail to make a distinction between people who eat red meat as hamburgers with fries and a large soda, and the relatively small number of people who eat red meat but also avoid processed foods and eat lots of vegetables. The ongoing health policy that demonizes meat consumption flies in the face of good evidence that a diet rich in animal fats and proteins is effective to control high blood sugar and elevated insulin,[7] the underlying factors behind the diseases that plague our society including obesity, diabetes, cardiovascular disease and cancer.[8, 9, 10]

Unlike rapidly digesting carbohydrates, proteins and fats are broken down much more slowly and thus release their energy over a longer period of time. In part this is due to a rate limiting mechanism called **gluconeogenesis**, which slowly manufactures blood sugar from proteins and fats, but only in response to the body's metabolic needs. In contrast, sugars derived from grains, fruits and sweets flood into the bloodstream immediately after digestion and provoke rapid alterations in blood sugar and metabolism. Compared to carbohydrate foods, meat and animal products are slow burning fuels that keep the body warm, stable and energized.

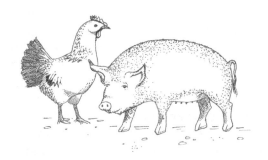

One major issue with animal product consumption is the reality that toxins have been accumulating in the environment for the last 200 years. Fire-retardants (PBDEs), heavy metals, fuels, solvents, hormones, antibiotics and pesticides are only a few of the many **pollutants** that are now found all over the world. Dispersed from regions of high concentration by water, wind and weather, these toxins accumulate within the food chain, and the higher up the chain the more concentrated they become. Even in what should be the relatively pristine environment of the Canadian arctic, very high levels of toxins are routinely found in the blood and hair of indigenous peoples eating traditional foods such as whale and seal.[11] Over the last 100 years the physical burden of these toxins has increased dramatically, passed on from generation to generation, concentrated in the fat of dairy, fish, poultry and meat, the problem now so bad that even human breast milk could be called a bio-hazard.[12] Given how these toxins accumulate in the food chain it makes sense to eat less meat, and indeed, some research shows vegetarians have lower levels of organochlorines in their breast milk,[13] lower levels of polybrominated diphenyl ethers (PBDEs) in their blood,[14] and lower levels of heavy metals such as mercury in their hair.[15] Nonetheless, it is important to recognize that the greatest risk of exposure to some toxins like PBDEs isn't from animal products but from house dust, derived from electronics, mattresses, furniture and carpets, accounting for up to 77% of our total daily intake.[16, 17] And while a vegetarian diet may reduce exposure to some kinds of toxins, other research suggests that vegetarians may be at higher risk of exposure to chemicals such as pesticides when compared to omnivores.[18]

The reality is that pollution affects everyone irrespective of diet, and while avoiding animal products may reduce exposure, in some cases the overall reduction may be statistically insignificant.[19]   If you decide to eat animal products it is important to choose organic, free-range sources. With regard to fish, shrimp and shellfish, avoid farmed species that tend to have significantly higher levels of persistent organic pollutants such as PCBs and PBDEs.[20] Certain species of wild fish including tuna, shark, swordfish, escolar, marlin and orange roughy may contain significant levels of **mercury** and should be limited to no more than 150 g per week; 150 g per month in breastfeeding and pregnant women; 125 g per month in children ages between 5 and 11 years; and no more than 75 g per month in children under the of age of 4.[21] When it comes to eating fish, I most frequently recommend small oily fish such as smelt and herring because they are lower on the food chain, and are particularly dense in vital nutrients such as vitamin D3 and omega 3 fatty acids.

Based on my research and clinical experience, the best types of meat, poultry and fish for regular and occasional consumption include:

- wild cold water fish, e.g. salmon, pike, arctic char, mackerel, sardines, pickerel, smelts/ooligan, herring
- organic, pasture-raised eggs
- organic, pasture-raised poultry, e.g. chicken, turkey, duck, partridge, pheasant, quail, emu, ostrich
- free range, grass-fed organic beef, bison, elk and venison
- free range, forage-fed organic lamb, mutton and goat
- free range, pasture-fed pork (including fruits, nuts and farm waste such as whey)
- wild meats such as venison, elk, caribou, and moose
- nitrite-free smoked, dried or canned meat and fish (mason jars)

In Ayurveda the classification of the different kinds of meat was often based upon the nature of the animal, in terms of its size or shape, it's behavior or habitat, as well as the properties of the meat itself. Generally speaking, the meat of dry desert regions is preferred over the meat of animals living in marshy, wet climates. And while meat and animal products in general tend to imbalance pitta and kapha, some types are less aggravating than others. Kapha tends to respond well to the meat of timid, quick-moving animals such as poultry, rabbit or deer, emphasizing leaner and drier cuts of meat. Pitta is balanced by eating animals that live in drier or cooler climates such as goat, elk, ocean fish and poultry, as long as they aren't too greasy in quality. Vata is balanced by most types of meat, and especially the meat of slow-moving animals raised in mild climates, such as beef, water buffalo, mutton or pork, emphasizing fatty cuts of meat.

One component of eating meat that is frequently over-looked is the traditional importance of organ meats, or **offal**, including the heart, liver, kidneys, tongue, thyroid, pancreas, gizzard, blood, testes, ovaries and brain. These foods are particularly dense in key nutrients, and were traditionally eaten as medicinal foods to support the health of specific organs. For example, eating heart regularly helps to strengthen the heart and cardiovascular system. Likewise, eating chicken gizzard helps to breakdown stones in the gall bladder and urinary tract. Liver provides a rich source of vitamins and minerals, and helps to support detoxification. Eating products prepared with blood such as black pudding and blood sausage provides an excellent source of vitamin D3. To treat impotence, Ayurveda recommends a milk decoction of goat testicle. While many organ meats find their way into supplements called "glandulars", the actual amount contained in these products is negligible when compared to food-based sources. While most organ meats can be eaten regularly, liver should only be eaten about once a week, as it it has high levels of vitamin A that could easily become toxic if consumed too often.

Please refer to Appendix V: Meat (p. 263) for a complete listing of their qualities, flavors and effects upon the doshas.

Cereal Grains

The defining difference between our native hunter-gatherer diet and the way we eat now rests upon our relatively recent decision as a species to subsist on cereal grains, most of which are derived from the Poaceae, or grass family. Instead of moving from place to place, following the migration of different animals, or to different climates in different seasons, agriculture allowed humans to settle in one place and grow most if not all of their food. Although our hunter-gatherer ancestors ate some types of wild grass, it was only ever a minor food and was never cultivated on the mass scale required to sustain a sedentary population.

As a species we have only been consuming cereal grains for the last 9000 years, which is a tiny fraction of time if we consider our two million year evolution as hunter-gatherers. Developing some time after the domestication of animals, agriculture spread its seed from places like India, China and the Middle East all over the world during the next several thousand years, only reaching some places in the last few hundred. Despite the global spread of agrarianism there is significant evidence that cereal grains fundamentally underlie much of the chronic disease experienced in human society.[22] As a disease of carbohydrate intolerance, diabetes is a particularly salient example – first described over 3000 years ago in the *Ebers Papyrus* of Egypt and the *Sushruta samhita* of India, two civilizations that had become increasingly reliant upon the starchy nutrition of cereal grains. Among the Greeks and Romans diabetes finds mention as a relatively rare disease but by the end of the Middle Ages and 1500 years of intensive agriculture diabetes is relatively common in Europe.[23] And in less than 150 years since being forced to abandon their hunter-gatherer ways the prevalence of diabetes among First Nations people in Canada has sky-rocketed to become an epidemic that is 3-5 times the national average.[24] Bolstered by history, more than two decades of research on metabolic syndrome and the link between elevated blood sugar and insulin resistance confirms that a reliance on dietary carbohydrates is an important cause not just of diabetes, but obesity, cardiovascular disease and cancer.[25]

Despite the problems associated with our reliance on carbohydrates, these concerns are balanced by the apparent virtues of dietary fiber. In contradistinction to sugars and starches, dietary fiber is associated with a decreased risk of developing obesity, cardiovascular disease and diabetes, as well as certain digestive disorders including constipation and hemorrhoids.[26] Comprised of indigestible sugars such as cellulose, fiber mediates the glycemic impact of carbohydrates, serving as a kind of mechanical barrier that slows the breakdown of complex starches into simple sugars. This property of cereals to inhibit digestion isn't limited to fiber, but is enhanced by a number of other compounds called **antinutrient factors (ANFs)**, including phytates, polyphenols, protease inhibitors, non-protein amino acids (NPAAs) and lectins. **Phytate** (phytic acid) reaches concentrations of up to 10% of dry matter in cereals and legumes, and functions to store phosphate and minerals required for seed germination. During digestion phytate forms insoluble complexes with a range of key nutrients such as niacin, calcium, magnesium, iron and zinc, minimizing absorption and leading to nutrient deficiencies. **Polyphenols** such as tannins similarly chelate minerals including iron and zinc, but also precipitate proteins and directly inhibit digestive secretions. **Protease inhibitors** block the function of protein-digesting enzymes such as trypsin and chymotrypsin, whereas **lectins** induce gut inflammation and may provoke autoimmune disease.[27, 28, 29]

Over thousands of years of experimentation we have learned to process cereals to limit the negative effects of antinutrient factors, including grinding, germination (p. 116), fermentation (p. 126) and cooking. While innovations in modern technology would have us dispense with many of these methods, history demonstrates that when we fail to observe traditional measures there can be dramatic repercussions. Pellagra arose as a mysterious disease in the South-Eastern US during the early 1900's, just a few years after cornmeal had been introduced as food to feed the poorer classes. **Pellagra** ravages the body causing skin lesions, chronic diarrhea and dementia, killing the victim in just a few years. It took almost 50 years before a scientist discovered that pellagra was caused by a niacin (vitamin B3) deficiency. Years later it was discovered that the traditional Aztec practice of processing corn with an alkali such as wood ash or lime (called **nixtamalization**) releases niacin trapped in the outer shell of the kernel.

While pellagra is now a rare occurrence, its underlying cause finds resonance in a whole new epidemic of gluten intolerance. **Gluten** is a naturally occurring protein found in the seeds of grass species including wheat, spelt, kamut, rye and barley. When ground into a flour gluten gives these cereals a glue-like consistency that allows the dough to rise, trapping the gasses released by the leavening agent like a balloon fills with air. Etymologically the word 'gluten' is derived from the Latin word 'glutinis' meaning 'glue', and it is perhaps no surprise that the sticky properties of gluten are used to good effect in other applications such as paper-making, wallpaper paste, paper-mâché and play-dough.

Given the sticky, glue-like property of gluten and flour it is easy to appreciate that gluten is very difficult to digest. At the extreme end are those who suffer from **celiac disease,** and exhibit a profoundly negative response to gluten consumption, manifesting characteristic symptoms including abdominal pain, steatorrhea, constipation and malabsorption. Although less than 1% of the population is diagnosed with overt celiac disease, researchers suspect **gluten intolerance** may be much more common than previously thought,[30] affecting up to 29% of the US population.[31]   Beyond the effect on digestion, gluten intolerance is associated with a number of other issues including:

- weight loss[32]
- anemia[33]
- fatigue[34]
- dermatitis herpetiformis[35]
- psoriasis[36]
- autoimmune thyroiditis[37]
- type 1 diabetes[38]
- uveitis[39]
- Addison's disease[40]
- infertility[41]
- inflammatory bowel disease[42]
- autoimmune liver disorders[43, 44]
- pancreatitis[45]
- peripheral neuropathy[46]
- dementia[47]
- epilepsy[48, 49]
- anxiety[50]
- migraine[51]
- fibromyalgia[52]
- arthritis[53, 54]
- osteoporosis[55]
- cancer[56, 57]

The typical advice given to confirmed celiacs and those suspected of gluten intolerance is to avoid gluten-containing foods such as bread, pasta, pastries, muffins and breakfast cereal. Gluten however is hidden in many foods, used by industry as an adhesive and excipient in processed and prepared meats, processed cheeses, condiments, sweeteners and candy, as well as breads "made without flour". Given its prevalence in the food supply gluten avoidance can be a difficult task for the consumer, especially outside of big cities and major centers, and itself can be a cause of chronic anxiety.[58]

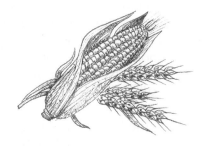

Given the association of gluten intolerance with chronic disease it is not surprising that the popularity of **gluten-free** products has exploded in the marketplace. Manufacturers have found clever ways to use non-gluten flours such as rice, buckwheat, corn, sorghum, teff, tapioca, arrowroot, potato, coconut, soy bean, guar bean and locust bean to make familiar products. While many of these alternatives do seem to lessen the symptoms associated with gluten intolerance, the question arises if we are substituting one problem for another. Very few of these alternatives were traditionally milled into a fine flour and used in baked goods, and many have the same types of antinutrient factors and immune sensitizers as gluten-containing cereals such as wheat.

It could be that much of the issue with the widespread gluten intolerance that seems to have evolved from thin air, like corn and pellagra, is in large part an artifact of not observing traditional methods of food preparation. Traditional methods of bread making, like the nixtamalization of corn, is an involved process that includes sprouting, roasting and stone-grinding the cereal to a coarse flour. The key element is the incorporation of a **sourdough** culture comprised of naturally occurring bacteria and yeasts. Apart from their use as leavening agents, these organisms ferment starches and produce enzymes in the process that effectively hydrolyze the gluten, turning it into easily digestible proteins.[59] Clinical research shows that when sourdough is used in the preparation of baked goods it is surprisingly well tolerated among patients with celiac disease.[60] Making *real* sourdough bread however is an artisan skill that requires time and effort to practice (see page 127).

While gluten-containing cereals may always remain problematic for some people, **non-grass cereals** such as quinoa, wild rice, buckwheat and amaranth are usually well tolerated. Among the grasses rice seems to be the best tolerated, and for at least half of the world's population is a word synonymous with food. To ensure good digestion, the best way to eat grains is prepared as a pilaf or cooked in soups and stews. While artisan sourdough bread made with a coarse flour is far better than any commercial product, it still maintains a sticky, heavy quality that makes it harder to digest.

Using traditional methods of preparation such as germination (p. 116), fermentation (p. 126) and roasting (p. 121), the best tolerated cereal grains include:

- quinoa
- rice
- wild rice
- amaranth
- buckwheat
- millet
- teff
- sorghum
- coix seed
- corn (nixtamalized)
- barley (contains a kind of gluten called hordein)
- oat (contains a kind of gluten called avenin)
- kamut, spelt, emmer, einkorn (all contain gluten)

In Ayurveda each type of cereal grain traditionally used in India is ascribed different properties. The most nourishing cereals are rice, oat and wheat, all of which are useful to balance vata and pitta, with rice tending to balance all three doshas. In contrast, barley is an important grain in Ayurveda to balance kapha, and is often the only grain recommended in the early treatment of diabetes. Most types of millet including finger-millet *(Eleusine coracana)*, Italian millet *(Setaria italica)*, proso millet *(Panicum miliaceum)*, kodo millet *(Paspalum scrobiculatum)* and sawa millet *(Echinochloa frumentacea)* reduce kapha and pitta. Wild rice, corn amaranth, sorghum, buckwheat and coix seed also reduce pitta and kapha. Like rice, the increasingly popular South American grain called quinoa balances all three doshas, and is an excellent source of protein.

Please refer to Appendix VI: Cereal Grains (p. 265) for a complete listing of their qualities, flavors and effects upon the doshas.

Legumes

Legumes are an adjunct to many traditional diets, and like cereal grains are products of agrarian civilization. They are derived from the Fabaceae family, formerly known as the Leguminosae, and contain a broad variety of edible species including soy (*Glycine max*), beans (*Phaseolus spp.*), pea (*Pisum sativum*), chickpea (*Cicer arietinum*), lentil *(Lens culinaris),* pigeon pea *(Cajanus cajan)* and peanuts (*Arachis spp.*).

Legumes are a good source of protein, and in a vegetarian diet helps to mediate the glycemic load of an otherwise high carbohydrate diet. Whole legumes are rich in fiber and can promote a healthy gut flora, assisting with problems such as constipation. Epidemiological research suggests that some legumes such as soy may have preventative effects in prostate,[61] gastric,[62] and colorectal cancer,[63] and may assist in reducing menopausal symptoms.[64] Leguminous plants are well represented in traditional medicine, and include many commonly used medicinal herbs such as licorice *(Glycyrrhiza glabra),* senna *(Cassia angustifolia)* and huang qi *(Astragalus membranaceus).* The Chinese herb bu gu zhi *(Psoralea corylifolia)* is a bean that is used to enhance fertility and as an adjunct in the treatment of psoriasis. The Indian herb kapikacchu *(Mucuna pruriens)* is similarly used to enhance fertility, and is a potent natural source of L-DOPA used in the treatment of Parkinson's disease. Like cereal grains however, legumes contain a similar array of potentially toxic or health damaging constituents including lectins, phytates and enzyme inhibitors, as well as isoflavones and non-protein amino acids (NPAAs). **Isoflavones** are unique to legumes and include compounds such as genistein, daidzein, biochanin A, formononetin and coumestrol that mimic the biological activity of estrogens, and hence are called phytoestrogens (i.e. 'plant' estrogens). **Non-protein**

amino acids are a group of protein analogues found in legumes that can have a wide range of potentially toxic effects including fetal malformation, neurotoxicity, dementia, hair loss, diarrhea, paralysis, cirrhosis and arrhythmia.[65, 66] Although traditional food processing methods such as germination (p. 116) and fermentation (p. 126) reduces antinutrient factors and NPAAs in legumes, the effect on phytoestrogens is less significant.[67, 68, 69]

Much of the negative attention on legumes has focused on soy, which is particularly rich in phytoestrogens such as genistein and daidzein. Called dadou, or the 'greater bean', soy has a prominent place in Chinese and East Asian history, described as one the five sacred grains (wu ku), used not only as a food but in crop rotation to fix nitrogen and improve soil nutrition. Although soy is frequently recommended to support healthy aging, one large epidemiological study found that soy accelerated age-related declines in mental function.[70] Other research has suggested a potential link between **phytoestrogens** in soy and male infertility[71] and reproductive dysfunction in women.[72, 73] And while dietary soy may have preventative effects in some types of cancer, soy protein isolate appears to promote the growth of estrogen-dependent tumors in a dose dependent manner.[74, 75] This is particularly salient due to the fact that soy protein isolate as well as other soy-based ingredients have become increasingly common in our diet, often hidden in foods we might not anticipate such as infant formula, processed meat, hamburgers, ice cream, baked goods, non-dairy substitutes, energy bars, snack foods, candy, margarine, vegetable shortening, mayonnaise, salad dressings and protein powders.

When soy made the transition from a cover crop to food in ancient China, it was never consumed without first being fermented, such as douchi (fermented black bean), natto, tempeh or miso, a process that deactivates antinutrient factors and enhances digestibility. About 1000 years ago the Chinese developed tofu or bean curd, made by curdling a soybean broth with gypsum dust – but there is no evidence that this properly denatures antinutrient factors in soy. Neither is there sound evidence that modern soy foods such as texturized soy (vegetable) protein (TSP/TVP) or soy "milk" are any better, even discounting the fact that most of the soy grown in North America is genetically modified.

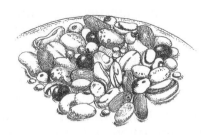

In Ayurveda legumes are considered dry, light and cold in quality, and thus all with the exception of urad (black gram) are contraindicated in vata (deficiency) conditions. As legumes weaken digestion they should be germinated (p. 116), roasted (p. 121) or fermented (p. 126), and then cooked with fresh water and spicy herbs. Gas and bloating is also a side-effect of eating too many beans at one meal. In places like India where legumes are a staple they are almost always prepared as a thin watery stew called dhal, cooking only one-small handful per person. Frying the beans in fat after they have been boiled is another practice that helps to balance out their dry, light and cold quality, practiced in India (e.g. dhal fry) as well as in other regions such as Central and South America (e.g. refried beans).

There are a large variety of legumes, and all have different properties and effects. Processing methods such as washing to remove the skins or splitting (e.g. split peas, split chana etc) does make legumes more digestible. This increase in digestibility however, sacrifices some of the purported benefits of legumes, such as fiber. As a general rule, I recommend whole legumes for healthy individuals, and split and washed legumes for people with weak digestion. The following is a list of what I have observed to be the best tolerated legumes and legume products for occasional or regular consumption:

- mung, adzuki, moth, urad, black-eyed pea
- chickpea (chana)
- pigeon pea (toor)
- lentil
- peas: dried green or yellow
- common beans, e.g. navy, pinto, kidney
- refried beans (homemade)
- fermented beans: black bean (douchi), tempeh, natto, miso, tamari

In Ayurveda legumes are generally indicated in both pitta and kapha to reduce inflammation, weight gain, edema and excess greasiness of body. Legumes are also indicated to remove wastes and toxins from the body, often prepared as a rice and bean soup (p. 180) that is used as the primary dietary article during detoxification (p. 209). The one exception to this general rule is black gram or urad, which is used to enhance fertility, boost breast milk production and promote weight gain. Urad is hard to digest though and is best cooked half and half with complementary legumes such as mung, and prepared with spicy, digestion-enhancing herbs (see p. 181).

Please refer to Appendix VII: Legumes (p. 266) for a complete listing of their qualities, flavors and effects upon the doshas.

Nuts and Seeds

Like cereal grains and legumes, **nuts and seeds** are a kind of fruit, but for culinary purposes are grouped into their own category. True nuts refer to a limited number of edible species with indehiscent fruits, wherein the seed or 'meat' remains enclosed in a hard outer shell at maturity, such as acorn, chestnut and hazelnut. In common use however, the term 'nut' simply refers to any oily seed enclosed within a shell, with 'seed' reserved for their diminutive counterparts, such as sesame or sunflower seed. Nuts and seeds are thus distinct from cereal grains and legumes by their higher fat content, even if from a botanical perspective the differences become a little confused. For example a peanut is a legume but because it has a high fat content is considered a nut. Likewise, an almond is botanically similar to a peach and is technically called a drupe, but because we eat the fatty seed inside the pit rather than the fleshy exocarp that covers it, we call it a nut.

Most nuts and seeds are rich in unstable polyunsaturated fatty acids and are thus susceptible to the negative effects of oxygen, heat and light. The best way to store them is in their hulls, keeping them in a cool, dry location. Once the hull is removed nuts and seeds quickly become rancid, developing a characteristic bitter taste. Nuts and seeds should have a sweetish taste, and if you detect any hint of bitterness it is better to discard the product rather than eat it. If you buy hulled nuts and seeds make sure they have been stored in nitrogen-packed containers, and keep them in a cool, dark and dry location such as the freezer.

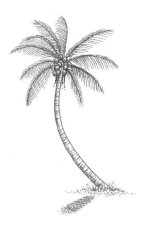

Nuts and seeds as well as cereals and legumes are susceptible to spoilage by fungi that produce secondary metabolites called mycotoxins, of which aflatoxins are a particular type. These **mycotoxins** have been implicated in allergy, immunosuppression, liver disease and cancer, and are the same class of toxins produced by molds that are responsible for 'sick building syndrome'. The growth of these pathogenic fungi is facilitated by humidity and warmth, and commonly affects nuts and seeds grown in warm climates such as almond, walnut, peanut, pistachio, brazil nut and cashew. One way to reduce exposure to mycotoxins is to carefully inspect the nut or seed for mold after shelling. Although this will eliminate specimens that are obviously infected, because the fungal hyphae and spores can only be seen with a microscope, it is by no means a foolproof method of detection. Industrial measures to reduce or eliminate aflatoxins include roasting, which damages heat-sensitive polyunsaturated fatty acids, and irradiation with materials such as cobalt-60, which remains a controversial practice. One way to significantly reduce mycotoxins at home is to cook nuts, seeds, grains and legumes in a pressure cooker, which has been shown to reduce aflatoxin B1 by up to 88%.[76]

Many nuts and seeds also contain a similar assortment of antinutrient factors (ANFs) found in cereals and legumes, which act to protect it until germination kicks in. A frequent recommendation is to soak nuts and seeds in water overnight to improve digestibility and remove pathogens, but while this does make them softer and hence easier to chew, there is little evidence to suggest that this alone is sufficient to deactivate anti-nutrient factors or mycotoxins. In traditional agrarian cultures nuts, seeds, grains and legumes were often fermented (p. 126) or germinated (p. 116) before cooking, which unlike soaking, results in significant reductions of ANFs such as phytate and protease inhibitors.[77, 78, 79]

Another way to reduce ANFs as well as mycotoxins in nuts and seeds is roasting (p. 121). Nuts and seeds relatively high in monounsaturated fats such as almond and peanut can be roasted in the oven at 320°F/160°C for about 10-15 minutes. To best enhance digestibility nuts and seeds can be added to grain dishes, roasting them at low heat with the grains in the pot for a few minutes before adding sufficient water to cook them (e.g. pp. 183, 185).

Once the inherent issues with nuts and seeds are taken into consideration, most can be safely included in the diet in small amounts, including:

- almond
- coconut
- cashew
- chestnut
- pinenut
- pecan
- walnut
- hazelnut, filbert
- pumpkin/squash seed
- sesame seed
- sunflower seed
- hemp
- flax
- chia
- peanut

From the perspective of Ayurveda nuts and seeds are the most nourishing (brimhana) foods of the vegetable kingdom, and are an excellent source of dietary fat (see p. 67). As the reproductive part of the plant, nuts and seeds are homologous to the sexual organs, and most such as almond, walnut, pinenut and cashew are traditionally used in Ayurveda to enhance vitality, virility and reduce vata. Nuts and seeds generally have a warming quality with the exception of tender coconut, which is used to balance pitta, reduce fever, ameliorate burning sensations and inhibit diarrhea. Some nuts and seeds such as hemp, flax, chia and sesame seed have edible fibrous hulls that readily absorb water, and can be soaked in water overnight and consumed the next day as a way to lubricate the intestines and prevent constipation. Due to their high fat content nuts and seeds can be difficult to digest, and when consumed in large amounts weaken digestion, aggravate kapha and facilitate the production of ama (toxins). As a general rule of thumb try to limit your consumption to only one small handful of nuts per day, and make sure to chew them well.

Please refer to Appendix VIII: Nuts and Seeds (p. 267) for a complete listing of their qualities, flavors and effects upon the doshas.

Dairy

Like the cultivation of cereals and legumes, the domestication of animals such as the cow is another feature of the Neolithic and agricultural revolution. Among the animals we evolved with the bovine genus seems admirably suited to domestication – a large powerful animal that can not only help to till the soil and pull a cart, but provides us with meat, leather, fuel and fertilizer. Among the gifts given to us by the cow there is perhaps nothing so valuable as her **milk**, a highly nourishing food, rich in all the proteins, fats and sugar needed for physical development. The classical texts of Ayurveda are replete with praise for milk and its various products such as yogurt, butter and ghee. The clear importance of milk in Indian culture is especially felt among devout Hindus who see milk as a symbol of the divine love that feeds our spirit, just as a mother feeds her young. Not just for providing milk but also for keeping the herd replenished and strong, the cow is both venerated and protected in traditional Indian culture.

Despite the great esteem with which Ayurveda holds milk, there is a growing trend here in the West to dismiss its purported health benefits. An increasingly large number of people are finding that when they eliminate dairy from their diet there is an improvement in their overall health. Sometimes the problem is associated with the milk sugar lactose, which many people lose the ability to digest as adults, promoting gas and bloating. In the baby calf **lactose** serves to increase gut permeability, thereby increasing nutrient absorption[80] – a feature that ensures the rapid physical growth of the baby calf, which achieves physical maturity in less than one year. This increase in gut permeability in humans however, most of whom regularly eat milk with other potentially immunoreactive foods such as wheat, may be among the different mechanisms involved in what is figuratively called **leaky gut** syndrome or **intestinal permeability syndrome**.

Apart from the issue of lactose, there is a significant amount of epidemiological evidence that links the consumption of dairy with the chronic degenerative diseases that plague agricultural societies, including acne, cardiovascular disease, diabetes, obesity, cancer and neurodegenerative disorders.[81, 82, 83] Many practitioners will attest to the fact that when dairy is eliminated from the diet their patients no longer complain of chronic symptoms such as sinus congestion, eczema, bloating, constipation, diarrhea and arthritis. Although calcium is often proffered as a reason to consume milk, there are many other excellent sources of calcium that are easily assimilated, including bone broths, almonds, leafy greens and sea vegetables. In my practice I regularly encourage people suffering from allergies, autoimmune disorders and chronic inflammation to avoid all dairy products except pure butterfat, i.e. ghee, which seems to lack the same immunogenic potential of milk proteins and sugar.

Much of the evidence against the consumption of milk has been accumulated in the last 100 years, during which time milk farming has gone from a simple rural practice to become a huge industrial operation. Normally fresh milk on the farm lasts about 1-2 days before naturally occurring bacteria ferment the milk sugars and cause it to sour. To prevent this, commercial milk undergoes flash **pasteurization**, a process in which the milk is heated to a temperature of approximately 72°C for 15-20 seconds, effectively killing the lactic acid bacteria. While this measure enhances shelf life it also causes damage to sensitive milk proteins such as beta-lactoglobulin and alpha-lactalbumin, enhancing their ability to provoke an allergic response.[84] Pasteurization also promotes losses in the nutrient content of milk, and deactivates the ability of raw milk to stimulate folacin uptake.[85, 86, 87] Perhaps most importantly, flash pasteurization does not completely sterilize the milk as most people believe, leaving behind heat-resistant bacteria that slowly putrefy it, causing the milk to 'spoil' rather than turn 'sour'. One recent study showed that pasteurized milk contains over 500 different strains of bacteria, with a general shift in the ecology towards the growth of *Paenibacillus*, an antibiotic-resistant bacterium that has been identified as a human pathogen.[88, 89, 90] Although more research is required, it seems very likely that this alteration in the ecology of milk facilitates some of the chronic health issues associated with dairy consumption.[91]

When fresh milk is allowed to sit the fat globules congeal and rise to the surface to form the cream, and when this is skimmed off it leaves behind the **skim milk**. In an industrial farming operation the milk is collected, refrigerated, pasteurized, cooled and then sent to a centrifuge to separate out the fat. The fat is then added back to the milk later to achieve a certain percentage (e.g. 1%, 2%, 3%, 18%, etc.). To prevent the fat from separating out again the milk undergoes **homogenization** by subjecting it to extremely high pressures between 1300-3300 PSI (10-25 MPa) in two stages: one to reduce the fat particle size by 400%, and then a second time to prevent the fat globules from congealing. This process fundamentally alters the structure of the fat globule, incorporating whey and casein proteins into its membrane.[92] Until the health effect of this alteration in the structure of milk is properly studied in humans, critics will continue to claim that homogenization is one of the factors that underlie the increasing frequency of milk allergies.[93]

Just like the diverse types of heirloom tomatoes or apple trees, so too are there a diverse number of milk-producing breeds, often perfectly adapted to the local environment. According to Ayurveda, different breeds produce different types of milk, and some are considered better for health than others. For example, the *Bhavaprakasha* states that the milk of a black cow is best to reduce vata, followed by yellow and red colored cows, whereas the milk of white colored cows provokes kapha.[94] In a similar vein, scientists have made a distinction between cows that produce one of two types of casein protein, either A1 or A2 beta-casein. Proponents claim that milk containing A2 casein, in preference to the A1 casein found in most modern dairy cows, does not have the same degree of immunoreactive potential as A1 milk, and is associated with lower rates of cardiovascular disease and diabetes.[95] What the cow feeds upon too seems to affect the overall quality of milk, with research demonstrating that the milk of grass-fed, pasture-raised cows has significantly higher levels of antioxidants, and naturally balanced ratios of omega 3 and 6 fats.[96] In contrast conventional milk from cows fed a corn-based diet displays very high ratios of omega 6 to omega 3 fats, leading to an imbalance in fatty acid consumption that research has linked to cancer, cardiovascular disease and diabetes[97] (see p. 67).

While it may seem that my position on industrial milk solidifies my support for your local grass-fed raw milk dairy farm, I do want to interject a small note of caution. There is a good reason why the government and regulatory agencies are concerned about raw milk. As I have attempted to illustrate, whether raw or pasteurized, milk is a living ecology. Without refrigeration raw milk at room temperature begins to ferment within a matter of hours, a built-in feature that we use to good effect in making clabber or yogurt. But it's a mistake to think that refrigerated raw milk is the same as fresh raw milk. Research has shown that when raw milk is refrigerated it suppresses the growth of lactic acid organisms in favor of pathogenic bacteria, with cell counts increasing dramatically in a matter of days.[98] These findings explain the occurrence of milk-borne disease observed among raw milk drinkers.[99, 100, 101] According to Ayurveda, while fresh warm raw milk straight from the teat is a health-giving food, raw milk that has been allowed to cool aggravates all three doshas, congests the channels of the body and promotes ama.[102] Thus to be perfectly safe I recommend that raw milk older than one day be prepared as boiled milk (p. 173), to be drunk warm, or be used to make cultured dairy products such as yogurt (p. 174) and cultured butter (p. 176). This is the way humans have preserved the health-giving benefits of milk for thousands of years. Just because industrial milk was invented doesn't mean that raw milk is unsafe, but by the same token, drinking cold raw milk right out the fridge may not be the health-giving food you think it is.

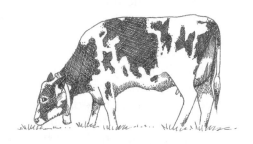

Ayurveda analyzes several factors when considering the benefits and disadvantages of milk consumption. Satmya is a term that refers to practices that are natural and normal to a particular person or group of people, and in the case of milk, suggests that it may not be for everyone. Although dairy is an accustomed food in many places there are some groups of people that do not traditionally consume it, such as among the Chinese or the First Nations people of Canada. Humans produce the enzyme lactase as infants but many people lose the ability to produce it later on in life, causing the typical lactose intolerance seen with milk consumption. This suggests that factors such as age or race can affect the suitability of milk in a particular person. Another factor to be considered with milk is the strength of digestion. Generally speaking, milk is heavy and greasy in quality and difficult to digest. People who consume milk should have strong digestion, and if not, the milk must be diluted with water and cooked with digestive-enhancing herbs such as cardamom, cinnamon and ginger (p. 173). Milk is also contraindicated for people suffering from the accumulation of ama, or autotoxicity, as the heavy and nourishing properties of the milk will also enhance the production of ama (toxins).

Ayurveda considers **cow's milk** (godugdha) to be cold, heavy and wet in quality. It is rejuvenating, nourishing, lactation promoting and gently laxative, alleviating vata and pitta but increasing kapha. Traditional texts describe that the milk of a black cow is considered to be the most wholesome, whereas the milk of white cow aggravates kapha.

Buttermilk (takra) is the acidic liquid separated from cultured butter during churning, and is considered to be cold in nature, stimulant to digestion and constipating. It is useful in the treatment of throat irritation and inflammation, but like cow's milk, is avoided in congestion and excess kapha. Buttermilk is especially useful in the treatment of dysentery when cooked with digestion-enhancing herbs, such as the traditional Indian dish called khadi (p. 177).

Goat's milk (ajadugdha) is similar to cow's milk in many respects, but is lighter in quality, easily digestible, constipating, and is particularly useful for wasting diseases, hemorrhoids, diarrhea, excessive menstrual bleeding and fever. Perhaps because goat milk is more similar to human milk than cow's milk, in many place in India goat's milk is the first choice when weaning children off of breastmilk.

Sheep's milk (avidugdha) is heavy and cold in quality, and is considered to be almost identical to cow's milk in action and effect. Sheep's milk is stated as being useful for pitta and vata conditions, as well as dry hacking coughs and hair loss.

Water buffalo milk (mahisidugdha) is very heavy and cold in nature, with more than twice the fat content of cow's milk. Given its rather gamey flavor, water buffalo milk is less preferred over cow's milk in India, and is most often consumed by the poorer classes. Water buffalo milk however is extremely nourishing, and is useful to treat wasting conditions, particularly when marked by a strong appetite. Water buffalo milk is also said to be constipating, enhances strength and is useful for insomnia.

When cow's milk is allowed to ferment the resultant preparation is called dadhi or yogurt (p. 174). Although high in beneficial bacterium such as *Lactobacillus*, yogurt can promote congestion and burning sensations, leading to fever, diseases of the blood, cold sores and other skin diseases. Fresh yogurt that is only a couple days old has a sweet flavor, and reduces vata and pitta, whereas really sour yogurt aggravates both kapha and pitta. Yogurt is good for digestion and helps build the tissues of the body. It is a useful remedy in diarrhea and dysentery, anorexia, difficult urination and in cases of chronic fever where ama has been removed (nirama jvara). Ayurveda stipulates that yogurt should always be consumed by itself, or with honey or jaggery, and never in the evening.

Panir (p. 178) is a cultured dairy product that very much resembles what we in the West know to be cottage cheese. It is typically made by curdling hot milk with an acid such as lime juice, and when the curds form, draining out the whey with cheesecloth, leaving behind the cheese. Panir is stated to be heavy, oily and cold in nature, and is a good food in vata and pitta conditions as long as the digestion is strong. Panir tends to promote congestion, and hence is a poor choice in kapha conditions such as excess mucus. Soft ripened cheeses such as mild cheddar, havarti and Monterey jack are usually very heavy in nature, and bear the same contraindications as panir. Hard fully ripened cheeses with a pungent flavor such as goat feta, romano or asiago cheese are typically well tolerated and don't produce congestion as easily.

Please refer to Appendix IX: Dairy (p. 268) for a complete listing of their qualities, flavors and effects upon the doshas.

Fats and Oils

While sweet foods like fruit most surely delight the senses, it is fair to say that what the body really craves is **fat**. Perhaps the reason is that compared to proteins and carbohydrates fats are a more abundant source of energy. With our comparatively huge brains, 60% of which are made entirely from fat, our evolution as a species can be defined by our drive to acquire this nutrient. Imagine if you were sitting around a campfire 200,000 years ago with an empty belly – what food would most satisfy your hunger? Sure, fruits and vegetables have their appeal, but if you don't want to spend all day chewing vegetation, what food fills your stomach best, and then gives you energy to do other stuff? Beyond any other food, fat was prized by traditional peoples all over the world, and as the rendered essence of an animal or a plant, was a kind of valuable currency that could be stored and traded for other goods. In Ayurveda, fat is the most nourishing of foods, and in Hinduism is equated with the goddess Lakshmi, the bringer of wealth, beauty and abundance. Everyday in India millions of people massage their bodies with oil to keep them youthful and healthy. Fat protects, comforts and soothes. Fat is like money in the bank.

Despite the traditional auspiciousness of fat there is perhaps no better example of a group of foods that have been so clearly targeted and maligned. Beginning in North America in the early 1900's, and then soon after in Europe and now spreading all over the world, industry and government have been trying to wean people away from their traditional high fat diets. Armed with an apparent avalanche of research reported on by the media, consumers have been led to believe that fat is killing them, regardless of the fact that the prevalence of our most common illnesses such as cardiovascular disease, cancer and diabetes have been steadily increasing since this marketing campaign began.

Even though this low fat marketing blitz that has permeated our fast-food culture for several decades now, the evidence for the benefits of eating a high fat diet is slowly being accumulated by scientific research. The difficulty thus far in validating the benefits of dietary fat is partly because research models continue to lump all dietary fat into the same category. For example, both French fries and herring oil are rich in fat, but clearly one will make you very sick if you eat it regularly, while the other is something humans been thriving on for tens of thousands of years. Often the claim is that the problem is saturated fat and cholesterol, and yet traditional peoples have survived for millennia on such fats. In China the traditional cooking fat has always been lard, and when researchers began studying this population, the Chinese people had lower rates of diseases such as diabetes when compared to Western countries. Flash-forward to modern times and now much of the Chinese population are using refined cooking oils – and sure enough – their disease rates such as diabetes are starting to match the West.[103] If saturated fat and cholesterol were ever truly harmful to humans, we would have died off long ago.

Also known as **lipids**, fats refer to a diverse range of chemicals including triglycerides, cholesterol, phospholipids, steroids, carotenoids, vitamins (A, D, E, K) and locally-acting hormones called eicosanoids. Like carbohydrates, lipids are comprised of carbon, oxygen and hydrogen, but the amount of oxygen in a lipid is much less, making for fewer polar covalent bonds. This means that lipids are insoluble in polar solvents such as water, but soluble in non-polar solvents like alcohol. This makes fats quite different from proteins and carbohydrates, and is the reason why lipids such as cholesterol must be bound to proteins such as LDL or HDL, in order to be transported in the blood.

When we speak of dietary fat we are referring exclusively to **triglycerides**, comprised of a three-carbon glycerol molecule that forms the backbone, and three (tri) fatty acids attached to each carbon in the glycerol molecule. The **fatty acids** are comprised of a chain of carbon atoms that have a variable size and shape, with hydrogen atoms attached on the side and at the end. When hydrogen atoms fill up every spot available on the carbon chain it is called a **saturated** fatty acid (a). When two adjacent carbon atoms form a double bond in the chain it is called **monounsaturated** fatty acid (b), i.e. 'mono' referring to the single double bond, and 'unsaturated' referring to the fact that the fatty acid isn't completely 'saturated' with hydrogen. A third type of fatty acid is called **polyunsaturated** (c), meaning that there are two or more (i.e. 'poly') double bonds on the fatty acid chain. The following diagram illustrates these differences:

a. saturated fatty acid, butyric acid 4:0

b. monounsaturated fatty acid, oleic acid 18:2Ω9

c. polyunsaturated fatty acid, linoleic acid 18:2Ω6

Structure of saturated, monounsaturated and polyunsaturated fatty acids

A given triglyceride may be comprised of different types of fatty acids, and so rarely is a fat completely saturated or unsaturated. The following chart lists common dietary fats and oils, and the different types of fatty acids each contains:

Fat type	% Saturated					% Mono unsaturated	% Poly unsaturated	
	Capric acid	Lauric acid	Myristic acid	Palmitic acid	Stearic acid	Oleic acid	Linoleic acid	Linolenic acid
	10:0	12:0	14:0	16:0	18:0	18:1	18:2	18:3
Almond Oil	-	-	-	6-8	1-2	64-82	8-28	-
Avocado Oil				7-32	<2	36-80	6-18	0-5
Beef Tallow	-	-	3-4	23-27	15-23	36-43	1.5-4	0.3-1
Butterfat (cow)[104]	2.1	2.6	9.4	24.1	10.9	28.2	2.1	0
Butterfat (goat)[105]	10	4.7	11.7	28.8	7.5	17.1	3	0.3
Butterfat (human)	0.6	4.1	7.3	25.6	7.9	26.8	10.9	0.5
Canola Oil	-	-	-	4.1	1.8	63	20	8.6
Cocoa Butter	-	-	-	24-30	32-37	31-37	2-5	-
Coconut Oil	5-10	40-54	15-23	6-11	1-4	4-11	1-2	-
Corn Oil	-	-	-	8-13	1-4	24-32	55-62	<2
Cottonseed Oil	-	-	<1	17-31	1-3	13-21	34-60	<1
Flaxseed Oil	-	-	-	4-10	2-8	10-20	12-24	45-70
Grapeseed Oil	-	-	-	7-10	3-6	14-22	65-73	<0.5
Hempseed Oil	-	-	-	6-9	2-3	10-16	50-60	15-25
Lard (Pork fat)	-	-	1-2	22-26	13-18	39-45	8-15	0.5-1.5
Marrow fat			1.8-2.5	23-26	15-18	41-45	2-5	0.5-2
Olive Oil	-	-	-	8-21	1-6	53-80	2-24	1-2
Palm Oil	-	-	0-15	22-46	0.5-5	36-68	2-20	<1
Palm Kernel Oil	3-7	46-52	15-17	6-9	1-3	13-19	0.5-2	-
Peanut Oil	-	-	-	18-13	1-4	35-66	14-41	<0.3
Poultry fat			0.2-1.3	22-28	6-11	37-53	9-25	<2
Safflower Oil	-	-	-	6-7	2-3	10-20	68-80	-
Sesame Oil	-	-	-	8-11	4-6	37-42	39-47	<0.5
Soybean Oil	-	-	-	8-13	2-5	17-26	50-62	4-10
Sunflower Oil	-	-	-	5-7	4-6	15-25	62-70	-
Walnut Oil	-	-	-	6-8	1-3	14-20	55-65	9-15

Common fats and their fatty acids[106, 107]

Saturated fats tend to be solid at room temperature and are commonly found in animal fats such as lard and butter, but are also present in plant oils such as coconut and palm kernel. Saturated fats are relatively stable and are thus a better choice for cooking and especially frying (p. 121). In comparison, dietary fats rich in monounsaturated fatty acids are more unstable, but certainly more stable than oils rich in polyunsaturated fatty acids, which oxidize quickly when exposed to heat, oxygen or light. One of the key issues that relates to fats is their role in the production of compounds called **eicosanoids**, including prostaglandins, leukotrienes, prostacyclins and thromboxanes. Eicosanoids are derived from linoleic and linolenic acid, two types of polyunsaturated fatty acids that the body cannot synthesize, and hence are called essential fatty acids. **Linoleic acid** is an 18-carbon fatty acid also called the **omega 6 fatty acid** because the first double bond is six carbons from the end, whereas **linolenic acid** is an 18-carbon fatty acid called an the **omega 3 fatty acid** because the first double bond is three carbons from the end. Linoleic acid and its active metabolite **arachidonic acid (AA)** are converted into a series of eicosanoids that tend to have a pro-inflammatory effect, whereas linolenic acid and its metabolites including **eicosapentaenoic acid (EPA)** and **docosahexaenoic acid (DHA)** tend to have an anti-inflammatory effect.   During our human evolution the consumption of omega 3 and 6 fatty acids was about equal, but with our relatively recent dependence upon cereal grains and vegetable oils in our diet and in animal feed, the ratio of essential fatty acids we consume has become skewed in favor of omega 6 fatty acids.   The net result of this imbalance is that we have a tendency to produce more pro-inflammatory eicosanoids, a feature that has been linked to chronic diseases including allergies, asthma, arthritis, cardiovascular disease and cancer.[108] Although our daily requirement for both omega 3 and 6 fatty acids is rather small, given that the average person consumes upwards of 17 times the amount of omega 6 relative to omega 3,[109] many practitioners recommend omega 3 fatty acid supplementation as a counter-measure.   There are issues with this recommendation however (see discussion under **fish oil**, below), and a more sustainable measure is to eat a diet that is naturally rich in omega 3 fatty acids, emphasizing pasture-raised animal produce, wild meat and fish, leafy greens, sea vegetables, and seeds such as chia and hemp seed.

Apart from the fats naturally found in the foods we eat, the fats we cook with must be extracted from their original source whether from animals or plants. The fat in milk called butterfat is extracted by first skimming off the cream, churning it into butter (p. 176), and then rendering off the pure butterfat from the milk solids to make ghee (p. 194). Animal fats including tallow, lard or fish fat are generally extracted by heat, such as boiling or roasting, and in industrial operations undergo further processing and refinement. Animal fats from poultry (schmaltz), beef (tallow), or pork (lard) can be rendered by carefully trimming the meat from the fat, and then slowly roasting the fat over an even heat (see p. 195).

The simplest method to extract an oil from a plant is the expeller press, which applies a mechanical pressure to express the oil. This low-tech method is used for many of the traditional vegetable oils we eat, from sources that have a high percentage of fat and are thus relatively easy to express, including olive (30% fat), sesame (50% fat), palm kernel (50% fat), almond (50-65% fat) and coconut (65% fat). The expeller process generally has a minimal impact on the quality of the oil, but under very high pressures temperatures can reach upwards of 120°F/49°C, high enough to cause some oils such as flax seed to oxidize.[110] In some cases the nut or seed is boiled or roasted before expression to render the oils more conducive to extraction, or in more recent times, non-polar synthetic solvents such as hexane are used. Such intensive techniques allow processors to express oil from sources such as grape seed (6% fat), corn (12% fat) and soy (20% fat) that are otherwise very difficult to express with an expeller press, and were never part of the traditional diet. Several of these newly introduced oils are sourced as by-products from other industries, such as grape seed from the wine industry, or cottonseed oil from the cotton industry.

While the expeller press typically yields a high quality product, when intensive methods of extraction are used the purity, quality and taste of an oil can be dramatically affected. As a result these oils require further processing, which may include degumming, neutralization, winterization, bleaching, deodorization (steam distillation) and hydrogenation. Some of these processes utilize chemicals and solvents to remove natural constituents such as waxes, gums, free fatty acids, vitamins and sterols. During **deodorization** in particular, the oil is heated to temperatures as high 446-500°F (230-260°C) for as long as several hours. **Hydrogenation** is a last step in which the oil is heated in a chamber with a metal catalyst and exposed to pressurized hydrogen gas. This is done to saturate oils rich in polyunsaturated fatty acids with hydrogen, turning it into a kind of saturated fat that allows it to be solid and shelf-stable at room temperature.

Hydrogenation is a process that fundamentally changes the physical structure of an unsaturated fatty acid, flipping hydrogen atoms across the double bond between two carbon atoms, changing them from *cis* ('same side') to *trans* ('across') configuration. **Transfats** have come under a lot of fire lately based on research that hydrogenated oils are associated with a higher risk of cardiovascular disease, diabetes and cancer. But 'transfats' are not the issue per se. In fact some transfats play a useful role in human health, like vaccenic acid and conjugated linoleic acid (CLA), both of which are naturally occurring in butterfat. More recently, researchers have linked trans-palmetoic acid, found in whole fat dairy products and meat, with a significant reduction in the risk of atherosclerosis and diabetes.[111] The label of 'transfat' obscures the real issue, which is the way industrial processing dramatically alters the structure of the fats we eat, removing essential fatty acids, vitamins and antioxidants, leading to nutrient deficiencies and gross imbalances in the ratio of fatty acids in the diet. Significant damage also occurs when oils rich in polyunsaturated fatty acids are heated during processing, altering their intrinsic structure as well as generating disease-causing lipid peroxides.[112, 113]

The following is a list of the best fats and oils for cooking, and the upper limit for cooking temperatures:

- organic butter: low-medium heat: 300°F/150°C
- extra virgin sesame oil: low-medium heat, 350°F/175°C
- extra virgin coconut oil (not copra): low-medium heat, 350°F/175°C
- organic lard or tallow: medium heat: 370°F/188°C
- extra virgin olive oil: medium heat, 405°F/210°C
- extra virgin almond oil: medium heat, 420°F/216°C
- organic palm and palm kernel oil: medium heat, 455°F/235°C
- organic (grass-fed) ghee: high heat: 485°F/252°C
- extra virgin avocado oil: high heat, 520°F/271°C

Note that I have not included many of the cold-pressed vegetable oils commonly touted as being a valuable source of essential fatty acids, including canola, walnut, pumpkin, hemp, flax, sunflower, safflower or perilla oil. Nor do I include essential fatty acid supplements such as borage, evening primrose and black currant oil on this list. While many of them such as walnut, flax and hemp seed are rich in fat, none were ever used as food oils since shortly after pressing they rapidly begin to oxidize, causing adjacent fatty acids to link together and polymerize. This makes them effective 'drying oils,' traditionally used in paints and varnishes to seal and preserve wood – but not as food. Apart from the damage that occurs to these oils during processing and storage, cooking these oils has also been shown to generate health-damaging lipid peroxides[114] (see p. 121).

To lengthen shelf life and preserve the quality of cooking oils, store them under cool, dry conditions. Even if a fat is naturally high in saturated fatty acids, factors such as humidity, heat, light and oxygen will all promote rancidity. Generally speaking, no fat or oil should be used for high-heat cooking.

Different types of fats have different properties, and traditional cultures have provided us with a detailed framework of what they are and how to use them. Fatty foods are typically reserved for people suffering from a vital deficiency, displaying signs such as weight loss, depressed immunity and weakness. Fatty foods are particularly useful for nourishing the brain during both gestation and childhood, to restore women after pregnancy, and in older people who show signs of wasting. In his excellent book on diabetes management, Dr. Richard Bernstein suggests that increasing the intake of fat upwards of 40% of the total caloric intake can be very helpful to stabilize blood sugars and insulin levels in diabetics.[115] In Ayurveda, fatty foods are typically avoided in the obese, in people with weak digestion, or in the presence of excess mucus, congestion or fever. Fatty foods (but not essential fatty acids) are also avoided in active multiple sclerosis (urusthambha), a disease in which the immune system attacks the fatty tissues of the nervous system.

Among the fats described by Ayurveda **ghee** is perhaps the most celebrated. Prepared from cultured butter (p. 194), ghee has a sweet taste and is cool, heavy and wet in quality. Balancing to both vata and pitta, ghee is considered to be a rasayana, helping to enhance and maintain vitality. Internally ghee is used to treat exhaustion, nervous system disorders and diseases of the liver. Topically ghee is anti-inflammatory and finds special utility in diseases of the eyes and skin, especially when prepared with bitter-tasting herbs such as barberry (*Berberis spp.*) and the Ayurvedic herbal formula triphala. Like honey, ghee is yogavahi, meaning that it contains the ability to augment the effects of any medicinal agent it is combined with. It is often combined with honey for its nutritive effects, but never in equal quantities. Although generally good for digestion, ghee can block the channels of the body and promote congestion if there is a lot of ama (toxicity).

Sesame oil (taila, gingelly oil) is another highly recommended food oil, and is the primary medium for the many different types of medicated oils used in Ayurveda. Sesame oil has a sweet flavor, and is warm, heavy and wet in quality, used to balance vata, enhance strength, nourish sexual function and clear the complexion. Applied topically sesame nourishes the skin and nervous system, helping to balance vata in the muscles and joints. **Coconut oil** is a fat frequently used in the south of India. It has a sweet flavor and a cool, wet and heavy quality, making it suitable to balance both pitta and vata. It is applied to reduce heat and inflammation, and to nourish and protect the skin. Most coconut oil comes from roasting the dried fruit (copra), which damages the integrity of the oil. Extra virgin coconut is preferred, either pressed from the dried fruit mechanically, or skimmed and purified from the fermented fruit. **Olive oil** and **almond oil** are both sweet in flavor, have a warm, heavy and wet quality, and are excellent to balance vata. Animal oils, including **lard** and **tallow**, are sweet in flavor and warm, heavy and wet in quality, and are useful for balancing vata. When used topically as medicated oils and salves, animal fats are much better absorbed, and are better carriers for medicinal herbs than vegetable oils. Among the different oils **marrow fat** is the most nourishing and balancing to vata; extracted from bones by boiling in water, cooling, skimming off the fat, and then reheating at low temperatures to remove any remaining water.

Fish oils, derived from fatty fish including herring, menhaden and ooligan (smelts), were exceptionally important foods utilized by many traditional peoples all over the world. They were typically produced by fermenting the freshly caught fish for up to two weeks, and then rendering off the oil by simmering at low heat in water. Rich in fat-soluble vitamins including vitamins A, D, E and K as well as omega 3 fatty acids, these rendered oils were not only an important dietary supplement, they were a valuable commodity for all coastal peoples, and were traded with interior peoples for other goods such as animal pelts and dried meat. In North America these 'grease trails' were extensive trading routes that extended deep into the interior, well beyond the Rocky Mountains, from Alaska all the way south to northern California. Recent scientific interest in the health benefits of fish oils has spawned a relatively new industry, and these oils are now found in the marketplace as a ubiquitous health food supplement. To meet consumer demand however, this type of fish oil is a highly refined product, and has undergone extensive processing to remove the characteristically fishy taste of traditional oils, as well as impurities and biological toxins. While there is research suggesting a benefit in consuming omega 3 fatty acids there is very little data on the effect that refinement has on the purported health benefits of fish oil concentrates. Rich in polyunsaturated fatty acids including eicosapentaenoic (20:5) and docosahexaenoic (22:6) acid, fish oil appears to be even more unstable than vegetable oil, and undergoes rapid deterioration under even optimal storage conditions, giving rise to health-damaging constituents.[116, 117, 118] Although there are clear benefits to eating oily fish, contradictory evidence raises questions about the stability of fish oil supplements if more than a month old from the date of manufacture.

Please refer to Appendix X: Fats and Oils (p. 269) for a complete listing of their qualities, flavors and effects upon the doshas.

Sweeteners

The decision to include a section on sweeteners is more a reflection of their great prominence in our daily lives, rather than my belief that they have any inherent importance in the human diet. This is not to say that sweeteners are not a part of some traditional diets, but that for the vast majority of our evolution we have not had access to them. Besides fruit the sweetest food our Paleolithic ancestors had was honey, gathered on rare occasions high up in a tree or off the side of a cliff. Our ancestors risked life and limb, not to mention the wrath of some very angry bees, just for the chance to taste it. Like fats and proteins have driven our human evolution, it could be argued that our desire for sweet represents the next phase of human civilization. But with sugar consumption linked to metabolic syndrome, and by extension, diabetes, cardiovascular disease and cancer, the problem with this new evolutionary trend is that it's killing us.

In essence all natural sweeteners are comprised of simple sugars like fructose, glucose and sucrose. Although naturally occuring, most of the time these sugars are locked up within tough, fibrous tissues and need to be extracted to get at their sweetness. The earliest agriculturally produced sweetener was most likely sugar cane grown in India over 5000 years ago. A member of the grass family, sugarcane resembles bamboo and grows in dense fields where it must be laboriously hewn from the ground with a large machete, and then bundled and carried back to the village. There the cane is broken, smashed and pounded to yield the juice, which is then subjected to heat, the liquid slowly boiled away over many hours to yield what in India is called guda, gur or jaggery. Given the time, labour and energy traditionally required to make jaggery, it is easy to appreciate how in ancient India sugar repesented wealth. Today in India, as it was in ancient times, sharing sweet foods is akin to sharing your wealth, and is often distributed to honored guests during celebrations such as weddings and religious festivals. Since the 17th century however, we have had the technology to take this nutritious food and extract the purest essence of its sweetness we call **white sugar**. In so doing we have created an extremely powerful drug; a white crystalline powder that is to sugar cane as cocaine is to coca leaf. In "emerging" economies like India and China white sugar has almost enitrely displaced traditional sweeteners, and as a result they have among the highest rates of diabetes prevalence in the world.

Not just cane sugar, but almost all the sweeteners we use are extracted on this same scale of intensive refinement. **Maple syrup** is rendered from the sweetish-tasting maple tree sap, but after boiling the sap down we end up with a concentrate that is roughly 50 times more potent than the sap itself. As an herbalist I routinely make herbal extracts, using ratios such as 1:2 or 1:3, and find such extracts to be fairly strong. But a 50:1 extract is out of my league, and has much more in common with a pharmaceutical drug. This issue also arises when we consider sweeteners derived from other sources such as sugarbeet, agave, corn, rice and barley, all of which must undergo the same degree of rigorous processing to extract their sweetness.

Regardless of its source, the drug-like properties of refined sweeteners cannot be dismissed. There is research demonstrating that sugar modulates the endogenous opioid receptors of the brain, with very clear evidence of physical withdrawal and craving.[119] In simple terms, this means that sugar has the same kind of effect on the nervous system as heroin – perhaps not as dramatic, but just as powerful. Just ask any heroin user and they will tell you that self-medicating with sugar is a natural way to prolong their high. The great irony is that we criminalize one type of addiction but then actively celebrate and encourage another. But whether it's shooting up in a dirty downtown alley or lining up for an ice cream cone at the local sweet shop, both groups of people are looking for a fix.

In Ayurveda, **honey** is viewed as the best among sweeteners, not just as a food but also as a powerful medicine that researchers are only now rediscovering. Simply put, honey is amazing. Collected as the sweet nectar from a variety of wildflowers and then regurgitated and concentrated within the honey comb for storage, honey is nature's answer to pharmaceutical extraction. Natural unpasteurized honey has been shown to display antimicrobial, wound-healing, antiinflammatory and antioxidant properties, validating the traditional application of honey as a medicine. The medicinal properties of honey as well as its flavor can vary to a large degree depending on which flowers the nectar is gathered from, such as manuka flower, honeysuckle, clover, fireweed, heather or orange blossom. In Ayurveda fresh raw honey is warm and moist in quality, but when left to sit for some time it develops a more drying quality. Overall raw honey stimulates digestion, dispels mucus, balances moisture, enhances the intellect and supports the sexual organs. It is used to balance kapha and vata, and in the treatment of cough, bronchitis, asthma, vomiting and ulcers. Externally, honey is used to heal bruises, soothe inflamed skin, resolve sores, unite broken bones and enhance the complexion. Like ghee, Ayurveda states that honey is yogavahi, meaning that it enhances the activity of any medication it is taken with. It is frequently used as anupana, or excipient, by mixing it with different herbs. Ayurveda however does prohibit the internal use of cooked honey because it may contain latent toxins that are activated through heating.

Apart from a similar intensity of sweetness, **jaggery (gur)** is very different from honey. Ayurveda states that this solid extract from sugar cane is cool, heavy and wet in quality, and is the best sweetener to balance pitta dosha, and is useful in the treatment of burning sensations and thirst. Fresh jaggery is soft and malleable like clay, but as it gets harder and dries out it becomes lighter in quality. Rich in minerals and easily assimilable nutrients, jaggery is used whenever there is weakness and malnourishment. It is avoided in kapha conditions such as congestion, mucus, obesity and parasitic infections including yeast syndrome. **Molasses** (organic) is the industrial by-product of sugarcane production, and has a warming and nourishing property that makes it a good food to balance vata and treat conditions such as anemia, fatigue and weakness.

There are of course many other sweeteners, and while all of them have slightly different flavors, because they are sweet and cool in quality they have similar properties and contraindications as jaggery. This includes toddy (made from coconut sap), maple syrup, agave syrup, barley malt and brown rice syrup. Non-caloric sweeteners such as **aspartame**, **acesulfame-K** and **sucralose** have all been developed in the last century, with evidence that some may be cancer-causing neurotoxins that have been rushed to market without sufficient research.[120, 121, 122] Low-calorie sweeteners including the sugar alcohols **xylitol** and **erythritol** appear to be safe, even if expensive, but xylitol in particular can cause gas and bloating. Natural-source non-caloric sweeteners include **stevia** leaf, **glycyrrhizin** (from licorice), **inulin** and **luo han** fruit. While it would appear that these and sugar alcohols are all acceptable alternatives to high-calorie and artificial sweeteners, just the taste of sweet has been shown to promote a cascade of neuro-endocrinal effects in the body that are indistinguishable from regular sweeteners, and may still promote undesirable metabolic effects such as appetite dysregulation and obesity.[123]

Tea, Chocolate and Coffee

According to Chinese legend **tea** *(Camellia sinensis)* was discovered accidently by the illustrious progenitor of agriculture Shen-nong when some leaves from the plant dropped into a pot of water he was boiling. Shen-nong was so taken with the flavor and benefits of this herb that he introduced the beverage to humanity, and as the legend goes, the Chinese have been drinking tea ever since. Spreading from China over the Silk Road into the Middle East, tea was brought to Europe by Dutch traders and then later the British introduced it to India. Poems have been sung about and wars have been fought over tea: it is a potent symbol of both sophistication and wealth, and in some cases revolution, appreciated not just for its unique flavor but for the benefits noted by Shen-nong millennia before.

The physiological effects of tea vary depending on the type and the person drinking it, but in general tea promotes both clarity and activity, stimulating both the mind and body. In physiological terms tea is a sympathomimetic, 'mimicking' or stimulating the 'fight or flight' or sympathetic nervous response. The active ingredient in tea is **caffeine**, complemented by smaller amounts of other methylxanthine alkaloids such as **theobromine** and **theophylline**. Collectively these alkaloids comprise upwards of 9% of the dry weight of tea,[124] but due to the high solubility of the mouth-puckering bitter tannins tea is rarely prepared as a strong beverage. As a result tea has an average caffeine content of about 40 mg, with much less for watery white or green tea, and upwards of 90 mg for strong black tea.[125] Although generally thought of as a stimulant, tea also contains a neuroactive amino acid called theanine (1.3%) that inhibits sympathetic activity, rounding out and balancing the stimulatory effect of tea.[126, 127]

Apart from its effects on the nervous system, tea also contains an array of antioxidants including flavonoids such as the catechins, kaempferol, quercetin, and myricetin. The catechin epigallocatechin gallate (EGCG) as well as other green tea catechins have attracted a lot of interest from medical researchers, showing promise in the prevention and treatment of cancer.[128, 129] Epidemiological research has shown that the regular consumption of green tea in particular is associated with a decreased risk of cardiovascular disease, and in general, promotes a longer, disease-free life.[130] Despite the health benefits of tea however, its regular consumption is not without some risk. Tea naturally accumulates potentially toxic amounts of both fluoride and aluminum from the soil, and is particularly concentrated in compressed ('brick') tea, oolong and black tea, with lesser amounts in both pu-erh and green tea.[131, 132]

There are several different types of tea, including white tea, green tea, oolong tea, black (red) tea and pu-erh tea. *White tea* is gathered from young and/or shade-grown leaves, wilted indoors and then baked to prevent oxidation. It has a mild flavor and a harmonious action in the body. *Green tea* is grown and dried in the open sunlight and then baked to preserve the green color of the leaves. It has a cooling effect, and is a good accompaniment to spicy foods or in symptoms of excess heat. In Japan the cooling effects of green tea are often balanced with roasted rice (genmai cha) that has a warming, nourishing property. *Pu-erh tea* is a type of green tea that has been allowed to ferment like grass clippings, which provides for a brown color and an earthy flavor, and is regarded as balancing and good for health. *Oolong tea* is allowed to oxidize awhile before it is heat-dried, and is considered to be more warming in energy than green tea, and is useful to hydrate the body. Oolong teas are sometimes blended with other flowers like jasmine, gardenia, magnolia, honeysuckle or rose to impart different flavors and effects. *Red tea* ("black" tea) is a completely oxidized tea with a dark red brown color, and has stronger, stimulatory effects, often used in winter to generate more activity and heat. *Bancha* or 'twig' tea prepared from the dried leaf stems has a harmonious, detoxifying action with little stimulatory effect. From the perspective of Ayurveda, all tea is light and dry in quality, acting to decrease kapha, while increasing both vata and pitta.

Most of the tea drunk outside of China is black tea, which due to its bitter and astringent flavor is usually mixed with lots of sugar. In India chai is a milky tea usually taken with several teaspoons of sugar whereas in the Middle East black tea is often sucked through a sugar cube or a chunk of rock sugar. In the United States most of the black tea is consumed as iced tea, which depending on the preparation, contains as much or more sugar than a regular soda. Wherever it has spread black tea consumption has significantly contributed to sugar intake and the worldwide epidemic of diabetes. Although black tea consumption is considered to be a vice by religious and spiritually minded people in India, taken without sugar there is nothing to suggest that a cup or two of weak black tea is unhealthy. Drinking tea with a little milk or cream also helps to deactivate tannins in the tea that might otherwise bind to and damage proteins in the stomach lining. As a beverage for regular consumption however I tend to recommend the traditional teas of China, including white, green and pu-erh tea.

Chocolate *(Theobroma cacao)* is an ancient food considered sacred by the Olmec and subsequent Mesoamerican peoples, with evidence of its cultivation as far back as 1100 BCE. Known by the later Aztecs as *xocolatl*, chocolate was an important economic and spiritual plant in Mesoamerican culture, reflected in its genus name *Theobroma* ('theo' – god, 'broma' – food). Chocolate was prepared by fermenting and roasting the seeds of the cacao pod, grinding them into a powder, and then beating this with water to create a bitter-tasting frothy drink. Compared to tea, chocolate contains much less caffeine (1.29%), but augments this with a higher theobromine content (3.35%), and given that chocolate is eaten rather than brewed as a tea, the stimulatory effects can be significant. This effect is complimented with psychoactive, mood-altering compounds in chocolate including anandamide,[133] phenylethylamine[134] and tetrahydro-beta-carboline alkaloids[135] that may explain the common use of chocolate to boost mood[136] and treat depression.[137, 138] Chocolate also contains polyphenols that have potent antioxidant[139] and antiinflammatory[140] properties that support cardiovascular health,[141] and may be helpful to prevent diseases characterized by endothelial dysfunction including hypertension, diabetes, dementia and pre-eclampsia.[142, 143]

Chocolate is not an indigenous food to India, and hence the traditional literature of Ayurveda is silent on its properties and benefits. Given its almost ubiquitous usage as a panacea among Mesoamerican peoples however, it is fair to suggest that chocolate is a health food, but only when used in its in traditional context. This means that most of the chocolate in the marketplace, which contains an average of 15% cocoa as well as numerous additives and preservatives, is a rather poor substitute for this 'food of the gods'. As a confectionary item the highest percentage of dark chocolate is a better choice, but can still contain very high amounts of sugar. Cocoa powder is also used as a savory ingredient in traditional Mexican sauces called moles, added in at the end of cooking. Raw cacao nibs are marketed as a source of antioxidant-rich polyphenols, but if they were truly raw it would ignore thousands of years of traditional practice, which utilizes both fermentation and roasting to deactivate antinutrient factors and mycotoxins in cacao.[144, 145]

Among the three prominent sources of methylxanthine alkaloids in our diet, **coffee** is the newcomer on the block. As one legend goes coffee, like tea, was discovered accidently, this time by a humble Ethiopian goat-herder rather than a celestial emperor. Another story is that it was discovered by a holy man named Sheikh Omar while he was exiled in the desert, later becoming a drink used by the Sufis, a sect of Islam that seeks to manifest a state of ecstatic transcendence through meditation, singing, chanting and dancing.[146] With Sufi monasteries becoming the first coffee houses, the beverage spread across the Middle East and by the 1600's made its appearance in Europe. Since then coffee has overtaken tea as the world's most popular beverage, doubling tea production by 6.6 million metric tons annually.[147]

Coffee only contains about 3.2% caffeine and very little theobromine or theophylline.[148] Despite this the solubility of caffeine in coffee is higher than tea, not least because it is ground into a fine powder before preparation to enhance extraction. The average caffeine content of coffee is about 100 mg per cup, more or less depending on the method of preparation. Espresso has lower caffeine content of between 58-75 mg per shot, whereas brewed coffee may contain over 250 mg per cup.[149, 150] As an essential method to bring out the different flavors of coffee, roasting also decreases caffeine content in the beans, with darker roasts such as French or Italian having less caffeine than medium roasts such as City or American.

Like tea and chocolate, coffee is another relative unknown in traditional Ayurveda, smuggled back from Arabia and planted near Mysore, India, by a Sufi named Baba Budan in the 17th century. According to the Arab physician Al Razi, coffee is hot and dry in quality, and has a stimulatory effect on the stomach.[151] From an Ayurvedic perspective coffee is warm, light and dry in property and is helpful to balance kapha. It promotes stomach emptying and stimulates bile excretion, inhibiting appetite and promoting intestinal movement. It is generally avoided in both pitta and vata, and should only be consumed after a meal, and never first thing in the morning. As a general rule of thumb coffee should be limited to 1-2 cups per day, as any more creates dependency and actively promotes other health issues including stress, gum recession, headache, bowel problems, arthritis, and back pain.

Maté or Yerba maté *(Ilex paraguariensis)* is another caffeine containing beverage from South America. Like cacao it has a long history of use among indigenous peoples and has become an increasingly popular substitute for coffee and tea in the West. Although sometimes marketed as "caffeine-free", maté contains about 2% caffeine and 0.5% theobromine.[152]

Alcohol

At the height of summer when the branches weigh heavy with fruit and the wafting sweetness saturates the air, the wild yeasts have already begun to feed. These ubiquitous fungi found on the skins ferment the fruit sugars to provide the yeasts with the energy needed for their growth and reproduction, and in the process, just happen to produce **alcohol**. Since these yeasts are everywhere, we all eat some amount of alcohol in our food, and thus consuming alcohol is as natural as eating. But while our hunter-gatherer ancestors no doubt ate wild fermented fruit, and maybe on occasion enough to get mildly inebriated, it wasn't until about 9000 years ago that we learned how to make wine. It perhaps has its origins in ancient China, but very early evidence of wine production has also been found in places such as modern-day Iran, a country that now forbids alcohol consumption. Not even considering the ancient Zorastrian culture of Iran, Persian literature is replete with references to wine, in the poems of Hafez and Sadi who speak of wine as a representation of divine bliss. From the drinking songs of college fraternities and sports fans, to intimate moments with family and friends, alcohol is a beverage of transcendence, as a way to leave behind our petty inhibitions and boundaries to share in the delight and ecstasy of everything melting away.

Wine has long been a part of Indian culture as well. In a 6th century Ayurvedic text called the *Ashtanga Hrdaya* two entire chapters are devoted to the subject of wine. The book outlines the properties of wine and its effects on the body, the dangers of overconsumption, intoxication and addiction, and how to prevent and treat these problems. Its author Vagbhata says that wine is a means to happiness, an elixir that brings about relief from the day-to-day monotony of everyday life. As the *Ashtanga*

Hrdaya says, "if he does not drink wine at least once, what else can he enjoy in this troublesome life of a householder?"[153]

According to Ayurveda, all alcohol has a hot and dry quality that quickly penetrates the tissues of the body, overcoming both the physical and mental qualities of inertia. In stimulating the body however, alcohol acts like a poison, catalyzing the innate vitality (ojas) towards forcible expression. With alcohol we become happy and joyful as this energy is released, but this loss also leads to mental instability, disordered thinking and impaired actions. The *Ashtanga Hrdaya* says that the improper consumption of wine is chief among the innumerable paths to self-destruction, leading to the loss of dharma (virtue), artha (prosperity) and kama (happiness).

Science supports the idea in Ayurveda that alcohol is a poison. There is clear evidence that consuming as little as two shots of distilled liquor, two glasses of wine or a pint of beer can produce liver injury when consumed on a daily basis. After consumption, blood alcohol levels increase dramatically and alcohol diffuses into the brain, producing the tipsy euphoria or buzz we get when we're a little drunk. The alcohol then passes through the liver where it is metabolized into acetaldehyde, which is highly toxic to both the liver and other organs, until it is acted upon by cellular antioxidants and reduced to acetic acid. Detoxifying acetaldehyde places great stress on the liver and interferes with normal functions, inhibiting gluconeogenesis and protein synthesis. It increases fatty acid synthesis leading to fatty liver (steatosis), in which the liver becomes enlarged and yellowed from the accumulation of peroxidized fat. This 'stagnation' of the liver is one of the major underlying factors of hangover, and is best treated with supportive measures such as antioxidant-rich foods, and especially bitter-tasting herbs, vegetables and fruit. While fatty liver is completely reversible, with chronic alcohol consumption the liver cells become inflamed (hepatitis) and eventually irreversible scarring (cirrhosis) begins to take place. Chronic alcohol consumption also induces a hypermetabolic state, increasing the activity of detoxifying enzymes, increasing tolerance to both alcohol and drugs, often leading to multiple substance abuse patterns.

To avoid these problems the *Ashtanga Hrdaya* prescribes a regimen for drinking alcohol, called **madyapanavidhi**:

- **Make sure you are in good health.** Alcohol is a kind poison that taxes the body, and if the body is weak alcohol consumption leads to further weakness and decline. In general, this rule refers to all intoxicating substances, but among them alcohol is prominent due to its particularly toxic effects.
- **Make sure you are in a good mood.** Alcohol may make you happy for a while, but if you were unhappy before drinking that state of mind returns before the negative effects of alcohol have worn off, leading to further unhappiness. In Ayurveda happiness is related to ojas – more vitality means more happiness. If you are using alcohol to change your mood, you might look for other things that give you pleasure and enjoyment first.
- **Make sure that you will be safe.** Ayurveda recommends drinking at home or a specific location, where you can't get hurt or hurt others, with "physicians" (i.e. sober people) watching over you. Travel is not recommended while drinking.
- **Make sure you are celebrating!** Drinking alcohol is a celebration, a sudden release of energy that is to be shared and enjoyed with good company and good food. Alcohol is particularly celebrated in the *Ashtanga Hrdaya* as an aphrodisiac, and some of the most suggestive passages of Ayurveda are found in its description of wine, and how we can enjoy it with our beloved.
- **Make sure to drink in moderation.** Have no more than two servings per event. That's enough to get pleasantly drunk for most people, and still not lose the ability to function. For more intimate settings the *Ashtanga Hrdaya* allows up to three drinks just to "please the wife"…
- **Make sure to take rasayanas after drinking.** Before retiring for the evening, take herbs that support the liver and build ojas. Examples include amla, peony, shatavari, punarnava, barberry, kudzu, turmeric, licorice and ginger, taken with honey, ghee or boiled milk.

Alcohol can be fermented or distilled. Common **fermented beverages** include wine, beer and mead. **Wine** is considered best for health, and because Ayurveda considers grapes to be among the best fruits, grape wine is the best among the different types of wine. At about 10-14% alcohol, wine (madya) has a sour taste and a hot, dry quality that stimulates the appetite, promotes circulation, benefits the heart and reduces vata and kapha. Red wine is richer in tannins, and has a drier and hotter quality than white wine that can aggravate pitta. Red wine is less likely to promote congestion and is best consumed in the winter and cold weather. White wine is more congesting and cooling in nature, better for pitta, and is reserved for warmer weather and warm climates. Wine can also be prepared with other fruits besides grapes, as well as with different herbs and flowers. In Ayurveda medicinal wines called **arishta** are used extensively in the treatment of a number of diseases and conditions, as they are also used in both Chinese and Western herbal medicine. Examples include *mustarishta*, used in Ayurveda for digestive problems; *shi quan da bu jiu*, a Chinese wine used to enhance vitality; and elderberry wine, used by Western herbalists in the treatment of colds and flu.

Beer (sura) has lower amounts of alcohol than wine, averaging from about 4-9% depending on the preparation. Unlike wine, beer is not good for digestion and tends to create congestion and weight gain. Rice beer (salisura) is considered to be the best among beers, whereas barley beer (yavasura) is considered inferior. In general beer is useful for nourishment and for promoting breastmilk production. Its properties also depend on the kind of herbs the beer is fermented with. In India beer was often fermented with a number of herbs including punarnava *(Boerhavia diffusa)* and bibhitaki *(Terminalia belerica)*, both of which are rejuvenating plants that are good for health. Today most beer is made with hops *(Humulus lupulus)*, a bitter-tasting herb with sedative properties that contains the estrogen 8-prenylnaringenin that alters sexual function.[154] In the Middle Ages men refused to pick hops because it made their testes shrink, and so hop-picking and beer-making became a woman's job. Each tavern produced its own unique blend of herbs to flavor the beer, some recipes using psychoactive plants such as henbane *(Hyocyamus niger)* and belladonna *(Atropa belladonna)* – hence the myth of the witch and the "devilish" effects of her cauldron's brew.

Mead (madhasava) is a kind of wine prepared by diluting honey with water and then either relying upon wild or added yeasts to ferment it. Unlike wine, mead is often flavored with different herbs, spices, fruits and flowers. Prepared simply, mead is light and easier to digest than wine, and is stated to be good for skin problems and urinary disorders. Like the medicinal wines called arishta in Ayurveda, a separate class of medicinal meads called **asava** are used for medicinal purposes.

Distilled liquor is prepared by boiling off the alcohol from a fermented mash of fruits, grains and just about any carbohydrate-rich food or alcohol. Examples include **brandy** (wine), **gin** (wine and herbs), **vodka** (corn or potatoes), **whiskey** (barley, wheat, rye, corn), **tequila** (agave) and **rum** (sugar). Distillation as a technique has been used in Ayurveda for thousands of years, and has long been used throughout the Middle East. Walk into any Persian grocery store and more than one aisle will be filled with different types of hydrosols, a distillate made from boiled herbs. Although distillation was known to the ancients, it was the Persian physician Ibn Sina in the 11th century that developed the refrigerated coil, allowing the distillate to condense much more quickly, speeding up the process of extraction. By about the 12th century the first evidence of alcohol distillation is found in Europe, and liquor soon begins to rival other traditional beverages. Oftentimes the variety of distilled liquor was marketed as a kind of medicinal tonic, such as gin made with juniper, an herb traditionally used to detoxify the body and enhance digestion. In the 19th century the continuous still was invented and distilled liquor production literally flooded the marketplace, giving rise to a host of social issues that sparked the rise of the Temperance movement and prohibition in North America.

Distilled liquor can range in alcohol content to anywhere from 30% (60 proof) up to 95% (180 proof), with most commercial distillates below 50% (100 proof). The higher alcohol content means that distilled liquor has a very pungent flavor, and a very hot and dry quality. It has a strong stimulatory effect upon circulation and digestion, and is an effective medicine to treat coldness (see p. 203) and reduce kapha. Distilled liquor is a suitable alternative for people with yeast problems (candidiasis), consumed dry, straight or with ice, as an alternative to fermented alcohol and sweetened beverages. Distilled alcohol however aggravates both pitta and vata, and should be avoided in warm weather and climates.

Section Two:
The Practice of Food

Diet and Dietary Therapy

A Short History of Diet

Human evolution has been a gradual process over millions of years, from our earliest ancestors that diverged from other primates over four to seven million years ago, to the modern *Homo sapiens sapiens* of today. We first begin to bear some semblance to the modern human as *Homo habilis* and *H. erectus* 2-3 million years ago, with rudimentary technology that characterize distinctly human behaviors such as hunting and gathering, using spears and stone tools, as well as the control and use of fire.[155, 156] The first anatomically modern humans known as *Homo sapiens* made their appearance as far back as 400,000 years ago in Africa, and over this time gradually developed technology and society until they began to undergo a radical transformation about 10,000 years ago. Collectively this period of time in archaeology, from the advent of *Homo habilis* to the agricultural revolution, is called the Paleolithic period, and represents more than 99.9% of human evolution.

As our primate ancestors evolved, the nature of our diet gradually shifted from eating plants and insects as tree-dwellers, to becoming the fur-wearing big game hunters that come to mind when we think of the archetypal 'cave man'. Out of necessity our diet was as diverse as possible, our ancestors maintaining a vast knowledge of local foods including plants, animals, fungi, and minerals in order to survive. Depending on factors such as geography and climate, how much of each type of food we might eat at any given time varied considerably. Researchers at the University of Colorado suggest that whenever possible our early ancestors preferred animal foods as their primary source of nutrition, comprising between 45-65% of their total energy intake, supplementing the remaining percentage with plant foods.[157] These findings corroborate evidence that suggests early humans preferred animal foods for its high calorie impact, a crucial evolutionary feature that allowed for the development of the characteristically large human brain.

About 10,000 years ago something revolutionary began to happen to humanity. Quite suddenly we began to experiment with the domestication of animals and plants, gathering together in settled communities to forgo our hunter-gather ways. The first wave of this happened in discrete areas in different parts of the globe: in Africa, the Middle East, India, China, Meso-America and Northern Europe. Whether caused by climate change, population pressures or some convergent mechanism of human evolution, our ancient ancestors began to leverage local resources to their advantage. Although animals such as the dog, pig and cow were among the first species to be domesticated, humans soon began to experiment with a diverse array of plant species, selecting and planting only the choicest specimens generation after generation, weeding out undesirable characteristics such as bitterness and fiber. The most outstanding feature of the agrarian revolution was the production and reliance upon cereal grains and legumes. Gathering, crushing, soaking, fermenting and cooking the seeds of various grasses including millet, emmer, einkorn, barley and maize yielded a surprisingly energy-rich food, while dried and boiled pulses such as lentil and pea provided a good source of protein. In the relatively stable global climate of this period, peoples that had already settled found that the reliable seasonal cycle of crop production yielded greater food security than the luck of the hunt, and slowly the foundations of human culture began to change. Gradually the diversity of foods in the diet began to decline as our Neolithic ancestors labored from dawn until dusk, limiting themselves to a few high-yielding species such as wheat and rice. Stored food became a valuable commodity in early human society, and used to advantage by a select few, helped to produce the social stratification we still see to this day, with an underclass of laborers and an elite that directs society by controlling food and its means of production. Since this time, although empires have risen and fallen, the diet of this toiling underclass has changed very little, at least up until very recently.

For your average peasant, poor hygiene, malnutrition and a lifetime of hard physical labor took its toll, but there was little evidence that they suffered from the chronic degenerative disease that is the hallmark of Western culture. In contrast, wealthy nobles that could afford the luxury of refined and processed foods, and were spared the labor and toil of an 'honest' living, often suffered from chronic diseases such as gout and diabetes. This stratification between the diseases of wealth and poverty continued more or less up until the "green revolution" of the 20th century. During this time industrial-farming practices dramatically increased food production, relying upon machinery, synthetic fertilizers and petroleum-based pesticides and herbicides to increase crop yield. Governments and corporations invested heavily in the development of new technologies to enhance the shelf life, flavor and preservation of food, altering the ratio of key nutrients in our diet and exposing us to a plethora of additives that we had previously never consumed. Within a few generations humble communities that at one time survived on subsistence diets were now eating refined foods formerly the preserve of kings and nobles. The impact of this change was observed by researchers such as Dr. Weston A. Price, meticulously documented in his book *Nutrition and Physical Degeneration*, confirmed later by researchers such as Trowell and Burkitt.[158] Less than a hundred years after Dr. Price published his observations, developing countries such as India and China that wish to model the economic success of the Western world have become afflicted with characteristically "Western" diseases, and now have the highest prevalence of diabetes in the world.[159]

The Paleolithic Diet

When we consider our 2-3 million year evolution it stands to reason that our bodies are best adapted to the hunter-gatherer diet of our Paleolithic ancestors. Although the assumption is often made that agriculture was in every respect an improvement upon the human condition, anthropological research shows that if our Paleolithic ancestors were able to survive accidents, infection and childbirth, their longevity was similar to that of the modern human, but without many of the chronic degenerative diseases that affect us now.[160] These conclusions are bolstered by contemporary research on the last few remaining Paleolithic groups such as the !Kung peoples of the Kalahari and Aché peoples of Paraguay, who are remarkably free of the chronic degenerative diseases that plague the industrialized world.[161, 162] The accounts of the first European explorers in North America are replete with references to the robust health and vitality of the Native Americans, who displayed little indication of the disease and pestilence the explorers left behind across the Atlantic.[163, 164] In the few hundred years since colonization and the adoption of the European diet however, Native Americans now suffer from the highest rates of diabetes, cardiovascular disease and cancer in North America.[165] From "robust" health to chronically infirm in just a few centuries, the Native American experience is only the most recent tale in the 10,000 years saga of our collective experiment with agriculture.

Cultivating a Paleolithic diet

The hallmark of the Paleolithic diet is an avoidance of agricultural staples including cereal grains, legumes, some types of nuts and seeds, dairy, refined vegetable oils and sweeteners. Although this apparently limits the diversity of the diet, many people are remarkably unaware of just how few types of foods we eat nowadays. Take a look in the shopping cart of your average shopper at the grocery store, and you will likely find the same five products such as milk, potatoes, wheat, corn and sugar. So while avoiding such foods may seem initially restrictive, it does out of necessity open up entirely new vistas in food previously unimagined.

- **Protein-based foods** on the Paleolithic diet include all pasture-raised, forage-fed or wild animal products, including meat, eggs, poultry, and fish (p. 45). Plant sources for proteins include nuts and seeds (p. 58) but as these contain allergens and anti-nutrient factors people with sensitive immune systems should approach them with caution.
- **Fat-based foods** include all fats naturally found in animal products, as well as the fat rendered from them including tallow, grease and lard (p. 195), and fatty vegetable foods such as coconut and avocado. Clarified butter (ghee) (p. 194) is not a Paleolithic food, but as it is rendered from sugars and immunoreactive proteins it is an acceptable food that rarely provokes a negative response.
- **Carbohydrate-based foods** include glycogen-rich animal tissues such as liver, as well as wild roots and tubers, wild fruits, and inner tree bark. In the Paleolithic diet I also include most root vegetables such as beets, rutabaga and Jerusalem artichoke as well as winter squashes and non-gluten grains such as quinoa, amaranth, rice and

buckwheat (p. 49), although very sensitive individuals may need to avoid cereals and legumes entirely (see Food sensitivities and allergies, p. 231). All non-starchy vegetables (p. 38) are acceptable in the Paleolithic diet with the possible exception of nightshades, including tomato, eggplant and bell peppers, which can provoke inflammation in sensitive individuals (p. 231).

- **Restricted foods** include gluten-containing cereal grains (p. 49), legumes (p. 55), dairy (p. 61), sweet fruits (p. 43), sweeteners (p. 76), tea, coffee, chocolate (p.79), alcohol (p. 84), and very starchy vegetables such as sweet potato, yam, potato, cassava, taro, dasheen and tapioca (p. 38).

The dietary ratio of proteins, carbohydrates and fats among Paleolithic peoples varied considerably depending on culture and geography, anywhere from 19–35% for proteins, 22–40% for carbohydrates, and 28–58% for fats.[166] One major factor missing from this equation however is the abundance of low-calorie non-starchy vegetation such as leafy greens, which are otherwise rich in trace minerals, vitamins and accessory nutrients. In my practice I suggest that when possible these foods comprise upwards of 50% of the total volume of foods eaten each to help to promote good digestion and moderate the appetite (see page 38).

While the Paleolithic diet may seem restrictive when compared to the typical Western diet, many people find that the immediate health benefits out-weigh the inconvenience. It is a diet that has low immunogenicity or allergy-causing potential, and thus people with food sensitivities and allergies often experience a lessening of symptoms when they have been on this diet for as little as a 1-2 weeks. Even environmental allergies such as animal dander or pollen lessen to the point of tolerance, and sometimes cease all together. With appropriate support this kind of diet can be very helpful in modulating the activity of autoimmune disorders such as multiple sclerosis and rheumatoid arthritis. In the treatment of chronic digestive disorders such as irritable bowel syndrome and Crohn's disease, the Paleolithic diet can be very helpful to lessen the reactivity of the gastric mucosa and normalize digestion. With its absence of refined carbohydrates the Paleolithic diet effectively inhibits fungal growth and development, and is useful to control chronic candidiasis (yeast) and related chronic fungal infections (e.g. rhinosinusitis). In the same way, the Paleolithic diet helps to normalize blood sugar and insulin levels, which in turn reduces the risk of diseases associated with insulin resistance including truncal obesity, hypertension, cardiovascular disease and diabetes.[167]

Although it is no miracle, the changes many people experience on this diet do indeed seem miraculous. In my clinical experience however some symptoms can actually worsen during the first few weeks of treatment, only to resolve some 4-6 weeks later. In traditional medicine this is described as a "healing crisis", and happens when the immune response shifts from a state of relative tolerance to an aggressive response that redirects the body back to homeostatic balance.

Please refer to Appendix II (p. 257) to review the Paleolithic diet meal plan.

The Ayurveda Diet

According to the *Charaka samhita* Ayurveda evolved out of a need to address the acute and chronic disease that emerged when humans first began to live together in settled communities. This suggests that the basic structure of Ayurveda could be as old as the Neolithic in India, some 10,000 years ago. By any measure Ayurveda is an ancient and venerable healing tradition, and has an enormous amount of empirical weight behind its practices, including diet. While I tend to recommend a strict Paleolithic diet in autoimmune disorders, obesity, diabetes and cardiovascular disease, the Ayurveda diet is suitable in many other conditions and as a general diet to promote good health.[168]

Ayurveda recognizes two basic diets: vegetarian and non-vegetarian. Each is chosen on the basis of a number of different factors including constitution, ancestry, climate, geography, season, age, gender and disease. Secondary factors include personal habits, aesthetics, religion and culture, although strictly speaking, these aren't within the scope of Ayurveda and in some cases may interfere with treatment. According to the late Dr. Mana Bajra Bajracharya of Kathmandu, a traditional Ayurvedic physician whose practice represented over 700 years of hereditary knowledge, there are prescribed ratios for each type of diet, whether vegetarian or non-vegetarian.

According to Dr. Mana, the general composition of a **non-vegetarian diet**[169] should be:

- three parts starchy foods (e.g. whole grains, starchy vegetables)
- one part meat, poultry, fish, or egg
- one part green vegetables and seasonal fruits
- one part liquids, such as herbal tea, water, etc.

Please refer to Appendix II (p. 258) to review a non-vegetarian meal plan.

According to Dr. Mana, the general composition of a **vegetarian diet**[170] should be:

- four parts starchy foods (e.g. cereals, starchy vegetables)
- one part legumes (e.g. dhal, beans, lentils) prepared as a soup
- one part dairy (e.g. milk, butter, ghee, curd)
- one part green vegetables and seasonal fruits
- one part liquids, such as herbal tea, water, etc.

Please refer to Appendix II (p. 258) to review a vegetarian meal plan.

The Ayurveda diet can also be modified on the basis of each dosha, emphasizing flavors and qualities in the diet that balance it (see Six Flavors, p. 23). Specific diets that relate to the doshas are only used on a therapeutic basis, to reduce and balance the aggravated qualities. In contrast, diets used to balance the constitution have a greater degree of flexibility.

Vata-reducing diet

A vata-reducing diet is predominant in sweet, sour and salty flavors, expressing the qualities of hot, wet and heavy. This includes foods such as:

- Soup stock made from bones, marrow and seaweed (e.g. Soup Stock p. 147)
- Nourishing, fatty meats prepared as soups and stews, e.g. pork, lamb, goat, mutton, fish, beef, bison (e.g. Five-Spice Bison Stew, p. 165)

- Leafy greens and other vegetables, eaten lightly stir-fried with warming herbs and spices (e.g. Spicy Saag, p. 154)
- Starchy vegetables, prepared with fat and moisture (e.g. Ginger-Tamari Winter Squash, p. 156)
- Whole grains and legumes, prepared as soups and stews with herbs and spices (e.g. Urad Mung Dhal, p. 181)
- Boiled milk, with herbs and spices (p. 173)
- Fermented foods, e.g. pickles, sauerkraut, kefir, yogurt (p. 159)
- Stewed fruits, prepared with spices and fat (p. 199)
- Nourishing oils and fats such as olive oil, sesame oil, butter, ghee
- Warming herbs and spices, e.g. ginger, cinnamon, garlic, fenugreek, basil, hing, cumin
- Salty foods, such as seaweed, sea salt and mineral salts

Pitta-reducing diet

A pitta-reducing diet is predominant in sweet, bitter and astringent flavors, expressing the qualities of cold, light and dry. This includes a preference for foods such as:

- Soup stock made from vegetables, mushrooms as well as cooling herbs and spices (e.g. Garden Vegetable Soup, p. 150)
- Lean cuts of meat, prepared baked or grilled, e.g. poultry, fish, bison, elk, wild game (e.g. Herb Poached Wild Salmon, p. 166)
- Leafy greens and other vegetables, steamed or eaten raw
- Whole grains and legumes, prepared as soups and stews with cooling herbs and spices (e.g. Goji Quinoa Pilaf, p. 184)
- Raw milk, fresh yogurt, buttermilk (e.g. Khadi, p. 177)
- Fresh fruit, with minimal citrus and sour varieties
- Cooling fats and oils, such as coconut and ghee
- Cooling herbs and spices, e.g. coriander, fennel, turmeric, clove, mint, cumin, licorice
- Cane sugar (jaggery, gur) in limited amounts

Kapha-reducing diet

A kapha-reducing diet is predominant in bitter, pungent and astringent flavors, expressing the qualities of hot, light and dry. This includes a preference for foods such as:

- Soup stock made from spicy herbs such as garlic, ginger, onion and chili (e.g. Mulligatawny Soup, p. 149)
- Limited amounts of lean meats, prepared baked or grilled, e.g. poultry, fish, bison, elk, wild game (e.g. Goat Curry, p. 169)
- Leafy greens and other vegetables, steamed or stir-fried with only a little fat (e.g. Garlic-Basil Rapini, p. 156)
- Light and drying grains such as barley, buckwheat, millet and wild rice (e.g. Northwest Wild Rice Infusion, p. 185)
- Most legumes, prepared with warming herbs and spices (e.g. Urad Mung Dhal, p. 181)
- Sour and bitter fruits such as lemon and lime
- Fermented foods, made with bitter and pungent vegetables such as onion, daikon, radish, cabbage, tomato, peppers (p. 159)
- Warming herbs and spices, e.g. ginger, cardamom, cayenne, ajwain, black pepper, mustard
- Honey, in limited amounts

Diets to treat more than one dosha are used in combination, eliminating the foods in each category that strongly aggravates a particular dosha (see Appendices III-X, pp. 259-269).

Vegetarian Diet

Vegetarianism is an approach to eating that limits or prohibits animal products in the diet, and can be of several different types including those that allow eggs (ovo-vegetarian) and/or milk products (lacto-vegetarian), or avoids animal products altogether (vegan). The practice of vegetarianism is relatively recent in human culture despite the reality that vegetable-based foods have always figured prominently in our diet. Sometimes the argument is made that humans are natural vegetarians but it is very clear over millions of years of evolution we have adapted as omnivores. We have a digestive tract that bears some similarity to carnivores, such as canine teeth and a stomach that secretes a powerful acid to digest proteins, but also the haustrated or pouch-like structure of our large intestine, which like the rumen of a cow is ideal for the bacterial fermentation of high-fiber vegetable foods. Our closest primate relatives including the bonobos and chimpanzees are both omnivorous, dining not only on leaves and fruits but also on insects and other small animals. Even supposedly vegetarian animals such as cows and sheep derive a good portion of their calories from eating insects naturally found in pasture and forage. If we look at it this way, we could say that there is no mammal that is exclusively vegetarian, let alone humans.

While there is weak evidence of vegetarianism in ancient Greece among the followers of Pythagoras, the wide scale implementation of a strictly vegetarian diet first comes to us from the sub-continent of India. The development of vegetarianism in India however appears to be relatively recent, with descriptions of animal sacrifice and meat-eating found in the earliest Indian texts such as the *Rig Veda* (c. 1500 BCE). Reference to meat eating and animal sacrifice are also found in the *Manu Smriti* ('Laws of Manu', 2nd century CE), which devout Hindus believe to contain the rules of proper conduct for their religion. The first injunctions against animal sacrifice are found in the heterodox socio-religious movements, including Jainism and Buddhism in the 6th century BCE. A characteristic of both these religions is that they reject the ritualistic imperatives of the Vedic religion, and instead emphasize a system of ethics based on personal action. Fundamental to both Jainism and Buddhism is the notion of karma, or the law of cause and effect. Both of these religions suggest that all human action initiates a cycle of corresponding reactions, and thus those who kill create a potential for their own harm, whether in this life or the next. Followers thus sought to sublimate this negative effect by living a strictly ethical life upon which was founded a respect for all living beings called **ahimsa**, or non-violence. For strict followers of Jainism, this means avoiding the consumption of any kind of vegetable in which the entire plant is killed, such as a root, as opposed to harvesting a leaf, fruit or flower, which does not kill the plant. This also meant not killing animals for food, although Jainism does allow for the consumption of milk since this does not injure or harm the animal. The most devout among Jains carefully filter out their drinking water to avoid eating any insects or microbes, and carefully sweep their walking path with brooms to avoid treading upon any living things. For Buddhism the practice of ahimsa extended to the killing of animals, but not necessarily to eating them. Thus as wandering monks that begged for food, the Buddha and his followers would eat meat if it were served, and would only reject the food if they knew the animal had been killed deliberately on their behalf.

The rise of these heterodox traditions within Indian society, and especially Buddhism which became the dominant religion in India for several hundred years, greatly influenced the later development of Hinduism. Ahimsa is mentioned as a central tenet in the *Yoga Sutra* of Patanjali (2nd century CE), and was propagated by the Hindu reformer Adi Shankaracharya (8th century CE) who built a new monastic order that was modeled after Buddhism. The practice of ahimsa also found resonance in the Bhakta movement in South India, which later spread through the subcontinent influencing Hindu practices and beliefs. By the Middle Ages vegetarianism had become a cornerstone of Hindu practice, aligned with the tenets of the *Hatha Yoga Pradipika* (c. 15th century CE) that recommends vegetarianism as a way to balance the mind and sublimate the passions (rajas) and inertia (tamas) of human consciousness. Today upwards of 42% of Hindus in India are strict vegetarians, with the highest percentage found among those born as hereditary priests (Brahmins).

As a practitioner of Ayurveda I frequently encounter the mistaken notion that Ayurveda advocates for vegetarianism, often in such a way that conveniently brings Ayurveda into the fold of the low-fat, high-carb argument expounded by some in the medical community. If one reviews the ancient texts of Ayurveda however, including the most venerable texts such as the *Charaka Samhita*, *Sushruta Samhita* and the *Ashtanga Hrdaya*, there is no mention of vegetarian foods being preferred over non-vegetarian sources. In fact, all of these texts make generous reference to the therapeutic use of a huge diversity of animal products, not only to treat specific diseases, but to maintain good health and vitality. While Yoga and Ayurveda are complementary, they are two distinct practices that have an entirely different focus and should not be confused.

Vegetarianism has only been practiced on a large scale over the last 2000 years, but despite this relatively short period of time Indian society has been able to create a diet that routinely produces healthy, long-lived vegetarians. There is reasonably good evidence that vegetarianism confers a number of health benefits, and when compared to people eating a conventional diet, promotes a healthier body weight, and may decrease the risk of heart disease, diabetes, arthritis, premenstrual syndrome, dementia and mood disorders.[171, 172, 173, 174] Some researchers have noted however that this benefit may be related less to an avoidance of meat than the increased intake of vegetable foods,[175] as well as the fact that vegetarians generally tend to exhibit a greater degree of health-consciousness than their non-vegetarian counterparts.[176]

Although vegetarianism has become increasingly mainstream in the West I am consistently surprised how few have researched the components of an Indian vegetarian diet, which would otherwise seem to be a pre-requisite. Apart from a diet necessarily rich in grains, pulses, nuts and seeds to supply the proteins and fats that are otherwise missing from a meat-free diet, the hallmark of Indian vegetarianism is the regular consumption milk and milk products. The importance of consuming dairy is clearly seen in the Hindu's veneration of the cow, which serves not only as an allegory of spiritual love, but provides a source of nutrients that are otherwise difficult to get in a vegetable based diet. Employing a variety of dairy-based foods including boiled milk (p. 173), yogurt (p. 174), panir and ghee (p. 194) not only provides for a density of fats and proteins unmatched by any vegetable-based food, it also provides vital nutrients such as essential fatty acids, calcium, potassium, magnesium and cholesterol that are difficult to get from a strict vegetable-based diet.[177] Beyond the ubiquitous presence of dairy the other feature commonly found in Indian cuisine is the diverse abundance of herbs and spices that not only enhance digestion to increase nutrient bioavailability, but contributes essential minerals and antioxidants that support health.[178] My recommendation for all who want to become vegetarian is to learn to cook Indian food, and the different ways to prepare dairy products, legumes and grains, and how to use herbs and spices. It doesn't mean that Indian food needs to be eaten exclusively, but that the strategies used to prepare and enhance the food are employed in a similar manner. To maintain optimal health I recommend following the established ratios of the vegetarian diet (p. 98) and use the meal plan on page 258 as a guide.

Veganism

Veganism is an approach to diet that eschews the consumption of any kind of animal product including meat, poultry, fish, eggs, dairy and honey. It began as a social movement in the 20th century that elevates food to both a political and spiritual consideration, with many adherents laying claim to the spiritual teachings of the East. Other advocates such as British philosopher David Pierce conflate the practice of veganism with transhumanism, the belief that humans can and should transcend their natural biological limitations. This thesis however runs counter to the teachings of Ayurveda, which states that human health is dependent upon our relationship with the earth and our ability to harmonize ourselves with natural rhythms and cycles.

While veganism certainly lays claim to high-minded ideals, the evidence used to bolster its position has some weaknesses. From an empirical perspective there is no reason to consider that veganism is a sustainable dietary choice, evidenced by the complete absence of any vegan culture in history. Even among the idealistic Essenes, whom proponents often claim were vegans, accounts given by Philo and Josephus suggest that the Essenes raised sheep and cattle for meat.[179] Similarly, arguments that veganism is represented in spiritual practices such as Taoism or Hinduism cannot be found, or are the product of revisionism and not the authentic traditions. Many proponents simply follow vegan dogma without doing the requisite research, repeating the same erroneous claims that humans evolved as vegetarians, or that our bodies are physically adapted to eating only plant-based foods.

While it is very true that a vegan diet is abundant in healthy foods such as vegetables and fruits, without rigorous supplementation it is also deficient in key nutrients including protein, omega-3 fats, cholesterol, iron, calcium, iodine, vitamin D3 and vitamin B-12.[180, 181] Among proteins, the vegan diet is deficient in important amino acids such as carnosine, a dipeptide found in muscle tissue that has been shown to suppress many of the biochemical changes that accompany aging, diabetes and neurodegenerative disorders.[182] One characteristic finding among vegans is what is figuratively called **failure-to-thrive** syndrome, manifesting as a pattern of complaints that includes chronic fatigue, poor sex drive, weight loss, impaired immunity, insomnia and constant hunger.[183] Research backs up the assertion that a long-term vegan diet impairs health, promoting weight loss, premenstrual syndrome and infertility,[184] impaired bone density,[185, 186] bone fracture,[187] dental problems,[188] and immunodeficiency.[189] A vegan diet is especially problematic and even dangerous in pregnant or lactating mothers as well as young children, increasing the risk of anemia, neurological disorders and developmental delay.[190, 191]

A vegan diet however is not without benefits, and can be a useful therapy to restore health, particularly in a society where over-consumption is the norm. Some clinical research has shown that a vegan diet is useful to control obesity and diabetes,[192, 193, 194] although it may compare unfavorably to more satiating high-fat and protein-rich diets that similarly promote weight loss and a reduction of associated risk factors.[195, 196, 197, 198] Perhaps the true benefits of a vegan diet may be in its ability to reduce the body burden of toxic compounds such as organochlorines[199] and other toxic compounds that bioaccumulate in animal products (see p. 45). From a traditional medical perspective a vegan diet is effective to reduce congestion (kapha), inflammation (pitta) and autotoxicity (ama), and may be very helpful when undertaken as part of a short-term detoxification program (p. 213) in the treatment of chronic disease. A vegan diet however is contraindicated in deficiency states (vata), marked by conditions including weight loss, fatigue, infertility, osteoporosis, and immune dysfunction.

Raw Foodism

Today there are an increasingly large number of people claiming that raw food is the best way to eat most or all of your food, informed by the theories of early 20th century advocates such as Edward Howell, Ann Wigmore and Herbert Shelton. Like veganism **raw foodism** has become a kind of underground social movement that equates social change with dietary choice. Broadly speaking raw foodists usually lay claim to one or two camps: those that only eat raw vegetable foods such as raw vegans, fruitarians and sproutarians, and the other that also or exclusively eats raw animal products.

Historically there are very few examples of raw food cultures. One notable example are the Inuit peoples, an aboriginal group of northern Canada called 'Eskimo' ('eaters of raw meat') by their southern Cree neighbors. While it is true that the Inuit do eat some raw fish and meat, the idea that they traditionally ate raw food exclusively is contradicted by ethnographic reports.[200] Besides the Inuit the only other indigenous groups that regularly eat raw meat also live in circumpolar regions, where frigid temperatures prevent against microbial growth and food-borne illness.

Raw foodism maintains several arguments, central of which is the idea that raw food contains vitally important enzymes that aid in digestion, and that by cooking food we destroy them. Taken at face value this theory seems to have a rational basis, but it doesn't account for the fact that the body produces far more enzymes in its digestive secretions than are found in the food itself. If it were true that these enzymes were necessary for digestion it would stand to reason that the body would not need to produce its own enzymes, when in reality the body produces up to five liters (1.3 gallons) of digestive juices on a daily basis. Like all proteins, enzymes are denatured and digested in the gut into their constituent peptide fragments, rendering them devoid of any significant enzymatic activity.

Raw foodism suggests that raw food has a higher nutrient value than cooked food, but what this fails to take into account is the issue of bioavailability. While cooking does reduce the nutrient content in some foods, it dramatically enhances nutrient bioavailability, offsetting any loss in nutrients by reducing the energy required for digestion and assimilation. According to anthropologists humans have been cooking food for more than a million years, and in the process have undergone both anatomical and physiological changes that reflect our reliance upon it.[201] Compared to our primate cousins, humans have a much smaller gut and yet characteristically larger brains (i.e. a higher encephalization quotient). Research suggests that cooking enhanced the efficiency of nutrient absorption, allowing for the evolution of a much smaller absorptive surface and hence smaller digestive tract, while at the same time boosting the energy intake required for the characteristically larger and more complex human brain.[202]

Some raw foodists also believe that cooking destroys naturally occurring microbes such as *Lactobacilli* that support gut health and prevent disease. Unless the raw food has been fermented to allow these "friendly" bacteria to out-compete other microbes however, raw food may also contain pathogenic bacteria such as *Campylobacter, Clostridium, Salmonella* and *Escherichia coli*. Other potential pathogens in raw food include pathogenic viruses (e.g. norovirus, enterovirus, hepatitis A virus), pathogenic fungi *(Aspergillus, Fusarium)* and parasites *(Giardia lamblia, Entamoeba histolytica)* that can cause both acute and chronic illness. In contradistinction to the claim that raw food is healthy, there are an estimated 76 million food-borne illnesses each year in the United States, accounting for 325,000 hospitalizations and 5,000 deaths, all from eating raw or improperly cooked food.[203] This is not to suggest that raw food is necessarily unhealthy, but that there are certain risks that need to be taken into consideration.

The last of the major arguments put forward by raw foodists is that cooking food results in the formation of toxins including glycotoxins, heterocyclic amines, transfats and nitrosamines. Here the argument for raw food finds its most strength, but much of this concern relates to specific cooking methods rather than cooking itself. In some instances raw food does have apparent benefits over cooked food, but these theoretical issues need to be weighed against empiricism and traditional practices. Although often couched in simplistic terms, the issue of raw versus cooked food isn't as black and white as many believe.

From a traditional medical perspective raw food can be eaten as part of a healthy diet but always with an eye to the nature of the food and the capacity of digestion. According to Ayurveda people that have strong digestion (pitta) can usually tolerate raw food on a regular basis, but consuming raw food all the time aggravates the quality of coldness in the body (vata, kapha), diminishing digestive activity and vital energy – a notion supported by anthropological evidence.[204] Although support for a raw food diet is weak in traditional systems such as Ayurveda and Chinese medicine, raw food has special therapeutic application in the treatment of disease and in particular to promote detoxification (p. 216).

Cookware

For the million or so years that humans have been cooking food we have relied on relatively simple techniques, such as cooking in a pit or over an open fire, using leaves to bake food in hot coals, or roasting with wooden grills, hot rocks and spits. Early **cookware** used by our Paleolithic ancestors included tortoise and mollusk shells, bamboo, hollowed gourds, carved stone and woven baskets. About 20,000 years ago we began to make crude ceramic cooking vessels made from clay, and as humans made the transition from hunter-gatherer to sedentary villager, our techniques became more sophisticated, incorporating other materials into ceramics such as bone, feldspar and quartz to achieve a harder and more durable cooking surface. Soapstone was also used as cookware during this time. Around 2000 BCE our ancestors began to work with and smelt metals including iron and copper, and gradually these were used in the manufacture of cookware. Up until recently, ceramics, iron and copper were the dominant materials used in cookware. Modern cookware materials such as glass, stainless steel, aluminum, silicon and plastic have all been developed in the last 120 years.

The most important factor to take into consideration in cookware is the cooking surface and how it might react with food during cooking and its overall durability. The following provides a brief review of the pros and cons of each type of cookware.

Ceramics

Ceramics include clay, porcelain and stoneware, and are among the oldest types of cookware. Compared to other cooking materials ceramics conduct heat rather poorly and must be heated up and cooled down slowly, otherwise they can crack. Although this makes them impractical for stovetop cooking ceramics are excellent when used to bake food in the oven, particularly when covered with a heavy lid to prevent evaporation. From a health perspective ceramics are very safe, but if they have colored glazes these may contain toxins such as lead, cadmium or cobalt that can leach into the food during cooking or storage. Porous, unglazed ceramics such as terracotta must be soaked 15 minutes in water before use, and are particularly good to keep the food moist during cooking.

Soapstone

Soapstone is an abundant mineral found all over the world and is comprised of talc as well as other minerals rich in silica, magnesium and iron. It was mined as early as 10,000 years ago, appreciated for its unique properties including its high resistance to heat, its relative softness for carving and shaping, and for its slippery, smooth surface. Soapstone cookware was used all over the world by ancient peoples in both Asia and the Americas; carved into various utensils including cooking stones, griddles, pans and pots. As other minerals readily migrate into soapstone its color can vary, from black and dark green to pink, pale green and grey, often indicating where the stone was mined. Today much of the soapstone cookware on the market comes from Brasil.

Soapstone provides an excellent, naturally non-stick cooking surface with very good heat conductivity. Due to the porous nature of soapstone the cookware needs to be sealed before using. After cleaning and drying, grease all the surfaces of the cookware with linseed oil (not boiled) and remove any excess. Bake the cookware in the oven at 500°F/260°C for one hour, and then slowly let it cool. Repeat the process one to two more times to get a nice non-stick coating. Like seasoned cast iron (below), make sure to clean the pan with water and avoid scrub brushes and detergents. The biggest problem with soapstone is that like ceramics it is quite brittle and cannot tolerate sudden temperature differences. For stovetop cooking make sure to use a heat diffuser to spread the heat evenly, and avoid thermal shock and possible cracking by slowly raising and lowering the temperature.

Soapstone has a very good safety profile, and any of the minerals that may migrate from the cookware into the food are regarded as harmless. The primary concern with soapstone is that it is mined in the same type of rock formations as asbestos. Due to the fibrous, brittle nature of asbestos it is unlikely to be found in cookware, but for absolute clarity ensure that manufacturers validate their cookware as asbestos-free.

Cast Iron

Cast iron is a venerable cooking material that date backs to the 3rd century CE in China, and became popular in the West during the 18th century. Although cast iron conducts heat rather poorly when compared to other metals, once it is heated it provides for an even and continuous distribution of heat. Cooking with cast iron does allow small amounts of iron to be leached into the food, particularly when exposed to an acid pH (e.g. vinegar, tomatoes, citrus). While iron cookware is helpful for people suffering from iron-deficiency it is best avoided by people with iron-overload syndrome (hemochromatosis).

To put them to best advantage cast iron pans need to be seasoned before use. Lightly coat the entire pan with linseed oil and roast in the oven at 500°F/260°C for 1-2 hours, repeating the process after the pan has cooled, applying a very thin coat of oil each time. Linseed oil has a special ability to polymerize at higher temperatures, becoming a kind of natural plastic that seals the pan. This then becomes the surface upon which a layer of carbon builds, and after many years of use, provides for an excellent (mostly) non-stick cooking surface. To clean, avoid the use of soaps and abrasives that can destroy the coating, instead using hot water and a cloth, leaving the cooking surface just a little bit greasy for storage. Cast iron pans are also an excellent and quick way to defrost frozen meat, often preferable to soaking in water, which can negatively affect flavor and texture.

Copper

Copper is another ancient cooking material that has excellent heat conductivity, but compared to iron is much more expensive and difficult to find. Copper also leaches into the food, but unlike iron is slightly toxic and is required by the body in much smaller amounts. Apart from the excellent heat transfer, copper pots have antimicrobial properties, which is one reason why copper vessels were used in ancient India to purify water. Nowadays most copper pans have been lined with stainless steel on the cooking surface.

Glass

Glass cookware is a relatively new cooking material made from borosilicate or tempered soda-lime glass (pyrex). Comprised mostly of silica, this type of glass cookware is generally non-reactive at normal cooking temperatures and very safe. It conducts heat well, but like clay and soapstone tends to be sensitive to rapid changes in temperature, and with improper use can shatter while cooking.

Stainless Steel

Stainless steel is an admixture of metals including iron, chromium, nickel, molybdenum and titanium to form a stain-resistant surface that inhibits corrosion. Stainless steel transfers heat better than iron, and although generally very durable, it has been shown to leach small amounts of metals into the food during cooking and storage.[205] The primary concern with stainless steel is nickel, which is a toxic heavy metal that can provoke allergies, and cooking with stainless steel has been shown to contribute up to 50% of our total daily intake of nickel.[206] Nonetheless the general consensus is that high quality stainless steel is a safe cooking surface, but should be avoided when preparing acidic foods, especially by nickel-sensitive people.

Aluminum

Aluminum is a very common cookware material owing to its excellent heat transferability, its light weight and low cost. Like all metal cookware aluminum has been shown to leach into food during cooking and storage, and for years there has been a concern that aluminum may play a role in neurodegenerative disease.[207] Anodized aluminum refers to a cooking surface that has been converted to aluminum oxide by electrolysis, and is generally non-reactive and fairly durable. Although there is little indication of any significant leaching into food, with regular use the anodized aluminum surface can become pitted and scratched, exposing the underlying bare aluminum.

Cheaper aluminum cookware is often coated with synthetic 'non-stick' polymers such as **polytetrafluoroethylene (Teflon)** manufactured by DuPont. While generally marketed as a safe, non-reactive cooking surface, there are many questions about its safety. The chemicals used to manufacture Teflon have been found to be bio-persistent carcinogens that bioaccumulate in the environment, and have been linked to cardiovascular disease, cancer and endocrinal dysfunction.[208, 209] At temperatures used even during moderate heat cooking, the Teflon coating has been shown to break down and vaporize, provoking what is figuratively called 'polymer fume fever', which is powerful enough to kill large birds such as parrots as well as cause lung edema and inflammation in humans.[210, 211] Teflon coatings also display very poor durability, and clearly wear off with cooking and cleaning. Although there is no independent research into the safety of ingesting polytetrafluoroethylene on a chronic basis, the material safety data sheet issued by Dupont indicates that long-term ingestion is associated with alterations in immune function.[212]

Plastic

Plastic is typically reserved for food storage, microwave use and counter-top appliances such as steamers, coffee machines and food processors. Research indicates that some of the chemicals found in food-grade plastics migrate into food during storage and heating.[213, 214, 215] Some of these chemicals, including bisphenol-A (BPA)[216] and phthalates,[217] are endocrine disruptors[218] suspected of playing a role in breast cancer,[219] prostate cancer,[220] obesity,[221] asthma,[222] neurobehavioural issues,[223] male infertility,[224] uterine fibroids and endometriosis.[225] While some manufacturers applaud themselves for no longer using chemicals like bisphenol-A (BPA), the fact that BPA was in widespread use for more than 50 years before its negative effects were realized, raises serious concerns about a host of other compounds in plastic that have not been adequately recognized or tested. Government agencies and industry continue to make confident claims about the safety of food plastics, but the reality is that this is an exceedingly complex field of research making it very difficult to generalize. Today research remains focused on the isolated activity of only a few out of the many different compounds found in plastic, and not their additive or synergetic effects. As a result, the net impact of food plastics on human health is largely unknown.[226]

Silicone

Silicone is a curious innovation in cookware, combining the flexible properties of plastic with a heat resistance of upwards of 425°F/220°C, often used in the manufacture of purportedly 'non-stick' baking pans and flexible cooking utensils. Despite its apparent safety, there is no data to suggest that silicone cookware is safe, but as guinea pigs to industrial design, consumers appear to be nonetheless destined to find out. Numerous rumors abound that cheaper quality silicon cookware products may contain fillers that could potentially leach into the food during cooking.[227]

In summation, the best cookware is made from ceramics, soapstone, seasoned cast iron and glass. Although still excellent for cooking, stainless steel, anodized aluminum and copper are my second choice. **Untreated bare aluminum, aluminum cookware with plastic non-stick coating, and plastic cookware, cooking utensils and packaging, should be assiduously avoided**. As for silicone, a lack of reliable safety data and as well as suitable manufacturing standards suggests that it should be avoided as well.

Food preparation

Raw

Raw food is food prepared without heat, and although the term suggests little in the way of processing, in fact the preparation of some raw food requires a significant investment of time and energy. With a few exceptions such as fruit and milk, nutrients in raw plant and animal products are trapped within fibrous tissues that we don't have the ability to digest, either because we can't easily chew it into a liquid slurry, or because we lack the enzymes required to break down materials such as cellulose. Some of the issue is aggravated by the fact that most of us fail to chew our food properly, but much of it also relates to limitations of biology and evolution (see p. 106).

Fortunately humans are adaptive animals, and raw foods can be rendered bioavailable by a number of different methods, using both simple and modern technologies. The simplest method of raw food preparation is to initiate the first stage of mechanical digestion by cutting, chopping, grinding or milling. Fruits and vegetables can be prepared as salads, chopping them into small pieces, and using herbs, salt and oil to enhance digestibility and nutrient absorption. Raw vegetable dishes can also be prepared with blenders, food processors and dehydrators to enhance digestion. Raw vegetable juice in particular is a powerful food for healing when used as part of a detoxification program (p. 216). Raw cereals, legumes, nuts and seeds also find their way into raw food cuisine, but should be at least germinated (p. 116) or fermented (p. 126) to denature anti-nutrient factors (see p. 49, 55, 58), and may need to undergo further processing by heat.

Raw meat, poultry and fish can also be eaten raw, in thin slices such as sashimi or ground into small pieces such as steak tartar or kibbeh, often mixed with herbs and spices as well as additional flavorings including wine or soy sauce to enhance absorption. Raw meat, poultry and fish can also be soaked in an acid medium such as lime juice or vinegar to denature proteins and enhance digestibility and flavor, such as the South American ceviche and the Philipino kinilaw. None of these methods however adequately protects against pathogenic microbes and parasites and as a general measure all raw meat, poultry and fish should be frozen to an internal temperature of at least -4°F/-20°C for at least 7 days before eating. [228] Fresh raw milk is usually safe (see p. 61), and raw egg yolk is also safe if care is taken to ensure that the eggshell is intact and clean before cracking it open.

Germination

Germination is the process by which a seed is transformed from dormancy into its active, growing form. A seed is comprised of three basic parts: the embryo, the endosperm, and the seed coat. The embryo is the vegetative part of the seed, while the endosperm serves as a source of nutrition for the developing embryo. The seed coat protects both in a tough fibrous outer layer. A seed is packed with all the nutrients it needs to begin the first stages of growth, and apart from the seed coat, is embedded with an array of antinutrient factors that protect it against microbes, insects and other predators.

When water penetrates the seed coat, it splits it open and activates plant hormones stored in the embryo. This in turn triggers the release of enzymes that break down antinutrient factors as well as the starch stored in the endosperm of the seed. The enzymes break the starch down into simpler sugars, which are used to support the growth of the first part of the seedling to emerge called the radicle, which forms the root. Later the plumule emerges to give rise to the stem and leaf structure. This explosion in growth during the first few days of germination not only liberates vital nutrients for the seedling but also dramatically enhances the bioavailability of these nutrients. Over thousands of years our ancestors discovered that germination was a key component to enhance the digestibility of cereals, legumes, nuts and seeds.

Germination is very simple and takes nothing more than the seeds, water, a big jar, some cheesecloth and an elastic band. Make a point to use whole grains and legumes to ensure the integrity of the protein-rich layer just underneath the seed coat, which contains the fragile enzymes required for germination. Place the seeds inside the jar and cover with water for 8-12 hours. Use the cheesecloth and elastic band to cover the opening and drain the seeds. Rinse well in cool water and drain again to prevent fermentation (p. 126). Put the seeds aside for another few hours and rinse and drain the seeds a few times a day, making sure that they don't dry out, but aren't sitting in water.

The constituents, energy content and flavor of the seed will change with the degree of germination. For most grain and legume dishes (p. 180) germinate the seed just until the radicle appears, or about 48 hours, in order to preserve the calorie content and starches. For vegetable sprouts keep them growing for another couple of days until the tiny leaves appear. While vegetable sprouts don't have as much food energy as sprouted grains, they do contain an abundance of vitamins and other nutrients. Sprouted seeds from vegetables such as broccoli, onion or garlic are good for a raw food snack or salad, but sprouts from cereals or legumes should be cooked (e.g. roasted baked, steamed, stir-fried) to deactivate antinutrient factors and lectins still found in the sprout.

Steaming

Steaming involves the use of hot water vapor to break down cellulose and other fibrous materials that lock up nutrients. After raw foods, steaming is the best way to preserve the nutrient status of your food. Different foods require different periods of time for steaming, and with practice, you will be able to steam any food to perfection.

The goal of steaming vegetables is to ensure that they retain most of their original color, but can be cut with a knife or poked by a fork with relative ease. Broccoli for example, when steamed properly, should be a brilliant green color, and yet be soft enough to cut with a butter knife. If left even a minute too long the broccoli will turn a drab green color, even though the consistency hasn't changed all that much.

There are various utensils for steaming, including metal mesh cages and bamboo steamers, or just put the food in a pot with a little bit of water and cover it with a lid. Avoid aluminum (p. 112) and plastic as these materials may leach toxic constituents into the food when acted upon by heat. When thinking about which vegetables to steam, include a variety with similar densities. Thinly sliced carrots and large broccoli spears, for example, cook very nicely together, but if the carrots are cut too thick the broccoli will be ready well before the carrots. Leafy greens such as bok choy, spinach and green chard steam quite quickly, as does sliced purple turnip, and should be added some time after other, denser vegetables such as carrots, sweet potato or winter squash. Beet greens and red chard are two kinds of vegetables that definitely should be steamed alone unless you don't mind all the vegetables having a bright pink tinge. There are no exact cooking times for steaming – just make sure to check frequently.

Salt is an important ingredient in steaming, and while it isn't always necessary, adding it facilitates the release of flavor and inhibits bitterness. This is especially important when steaming coarser leafy greens such as kale and cabbage, which benefit from a little salt to help penetrate the tough fibers while steaming.

One of the nicest features of steamed foods is that all of the natural flavors of the food come alive. When I steam my food, I rarely use a condiment, or if I do, such as a little black pepper, garlic butter or rosemary olive oil, it only serves to enhance the original flavor. When I've been eating a lot of heavily flavored foods I crave the crisp and pure flavor of steamed vegetables. Steamed vegetables are often a good way to get children to eat vegetables, particularly when introduced while young. When my children were small we would only serve steamed vegetables on their plate, and only when they ate these did we serve the remainder of the meal. To this day the steaming pile of veggies are the first thing to disappear from their plates.

Some animal foods are excellent when steamed or poached, such as the light meats including poultry and fish. Although rather bland on their own, fish and chicken are easily complemented with ingredients such as white wine, celery, shallots, crushed fresh garlic, chopped chives, rosemary, oregano, dill, salt and black pepper. Or try Asian style with a little sherry, grated ginger, tamari, toasted sesame oil and chopped cilantro. The variations are endless.

Boiling, Stewing and Braising

Boiling, stewing and braising are all similar to steaming except that instead of water vapor to break down the food, these methods require immersion in liquid. They are particularly suited for foods that are very dense, such as root vegetables, or are dehydrated and hard, and require immersion in hot water to soften them up, such as grains and legumes.

Some animal foods are best prepared by **boiling**, such as clams, mussels and crustaceans, and to flavor the food the boiling water can contain various ingredients such as celery, shallots, wine and herbs. For most other foods however continuous boiling is a rather severe process, and so once the water is brought to a boil the heat is reduced to a simmer, and a lid used to moderate the rate of evaporation. As opposed to boiling, the process of **stewing** allows the immersed food to slowly become penetrated by the water, preventing changes in the structure of the food that result in toughness, particularly with meat. At the same time, nutrients are liberated from the food into the fluid or broth to make a stock (p. 147).

Braising is essentially no different from stewing, and is an excellent way to prepare cuts of meat that are otherwise too tough to fry or bake, such as brisket and shanks. In both Ayurveda and Chinese medicine soups and stews prepared by this method are augmented with medicinal herbs to create delicious dishes that have a special ability to prevent and treat disease. Braising can be achieved by using both stovetop and oven methods to yield a very similar result. Glass, ceramics, and ceramic-lined cast iron cookware fitted with a heavy lid are excellent options for braising in the oven. Stovetop braising is also possible, but because the heat source is only applied from the bottom it may require stirring and can take a little longer. One way to speed this process up is to use a pressure cooker. While sometimes maligned as dangerous, modern pressure-cookers fitted with silicon gaskets are very safe and can be used to prepare healthy traditional dishes that normally take many hours of preparation in under an hour, effectively preserving nutrients while reducing energy costs by up to 70%.[229, 230]

Baking and Roasting

Baking and roasting is the use of dry heat to cook food, using the principle of convection rather than direct radiation (e.g. frying, grilling). It is a particularly good method to decrease the moisture of the food, essentially dehydrating it. Some foods benefit from this process such as bread that loses its moisture through baking to form a solid loaf. Other foods such as meat or vegetables however can easily become too dehydrated and rather tough and unappealing in the process. When determining what food you should bake or roast versus other methods of cooking, reserve this method for foods that have a high moisture content or contain a significant amount of fat.

Baking and roasting are highly effective for releasing and modifying aromatic principles contained in the food, such as the characteristic odor of baking bread. The underlying chemical process is called the **Maillard reaction**, a chemical reaction between an amino acid and a sugar under the influence of heat, creating a number of chemical derivatives that are responsible for a wide-range of flavors, depending on the type of amino acids involved. Maillard reactions are harnessed by the food and beverage flavoring industry, in the synthesis of artificial flavorings. Foods rich in carbohydrates also undergo caramelization, a process that relates only to the oxidation of sugars and not amino acids, yielding a characteristic nutty flavor.

While baking and roasting are useful methods to enhance the flavor of food, the very production of these flavors through the Maillard reaction also produces a number of secondary compounds such as glycotoxins and acrylamide. **Glycotoxins**, or **advanced glycosylation end-products (AGEs)**, have been linked to chronic inflammation, diabetes, cardiovascular disease and neurodegeneration, and are a major mechanism of aging including wrinkled skin.[231, 232] **Acrylamide** is a suspected carcinogen that is produced exclusively from starchy foods such as cereal grains and potato during baking or deep-frying.[233] The amount of glycotoxins and acrylamide increases with longer cooking times and higher temperatures, and so it is important not to cook food too long nor use too high a heat. A general rule of thumb is to avoid eating any cooked food that has a color beyond golden-brown, i.e. is dark brown, burnt or blackened. A craving for burned or blackened food is called 'pica' in the medical literature and could be a sign of a mineral deficiency such as iron.

Besides favorites such as leg of lamb and chicken, the most common food I bake or roast are root vegetables and squashes, usually in a baking dish with a lid to speed cooking time and to avoid any charring of the starches. In this way a delicious medley of foods can be cooked together including sweet potatoes, new potatoes, parsnips and winter squash, doused with olive oil and tossed with herbs and spices such as garlic, basil, rosemary, oregano, salt and pepper. It is an ideal cooking method when you are pressed for time, have lots to do, or are busy cooking other dishes. Just throw all these foods and flavors into a baking dish, cover with a lid, turn the oven up to about 175°C (350 °F), and in 45 minutes to an hour you have a delightful and nutritious accompaniment to almost any meal.

Roasting and antinutrients

Roasting is another way to reduce antinutrient factors (ANFs) in cereals, legumes, nuts and seeds. This can be done after germination when preparing a flour to make bread, or in the pot before adding water when making a boiled grain dish. Make sure to use a low-medium heat so as not to damage the fats. Nuts and seeds rich in polyunsaturated fats such as walnut, sunflower, flax or hemp should not be roasted at all. If preparing a flour from germinated cereals or legumes (p. 116), drain the sprouted grains and spread out onto some cookie sheets. Roast the sprouted cereal or legume in the oven at low heat (150°F/65°C) until dry, or about 6-8 hours, stirring periodically. Allow to cool, then grind into a flour.

Frying

Among the different cooking methods frying gets the most negative attention, simply because of our conditioned fear around the purported dangers of fat. Once we realize that many of these fears are unfounded, provided you follow some basic rules, you can confidently continue to fry your food.

Frying involves the use of fat and heat to cook the food, the heated oil preventing the food from sticking to the pan, as well as permeating the tissues of the food to break down fibers and render nutrients bioavailable. Frying also helps to spread and mix the flavors of the food, as many of the flavor compounds are soluble in fat. A general rule of thumb followed by all chefs is that flavor follows the fat, in much the same manner as the constituents of herbs are transferred to the oil when making a medicated herbal oil or salve.

When oils are exposed to heat they are subject to degradation through a process called **lipid peroxidation** in which a heat-generated free radical turns a fatty acid into a lipid peroxide. Once activated this lipid peroxide attacks an adjacent fatty acid, initiating a chain-reaction that only terminates when the pool of fatty acids is largely exhausted, or is inhibited by antioxidants such as vitamin E. All human cells are surrounded by fatty acids that form the plasma membrane, and a disruption to the integrity of the cell membrane through lipid peroxidation results in cell damage. The process of lipid peroxidation also results in the production of highly toxic **advanced lipoxidation end products (ALEs)** such as malondialdehyde and 4-hydroxynonenal (HNE). Like the glycotoxins mentioned under baking and roasting (p. 119), ALEs result in damage to cellular proteins and DNA, and are associated with chronic inflammation, neurodegeneration, cardiovascular disease, diabetes, and cancer.[234]

While all fats are subject to the effects of heat and the generation of free radicals during cooking, saturated fats are completely 'filled up' with hydrogen atoms and are relatively resistant to oxidation. In contrast, monounsaturated fats have one double bond susceptible to oxidation, whereas polyunsaturated fats have multiple double bonds making them highly vulnerable to peroxidation. Fats rich in saturated fatty acids like ghee and avocado oil are thus better for cooking, up to temperatures of 450°F/232°C. Fats rich in monounsaturated fatty acids such as lard, tallow, olive and almond oil can be used for medium heat cooking, up to a maximum temperature of 375°F/191°C. Fats rich in polyunsaturated fatty acids such as safflower, walnut, sunflower, flax or hemp are highly unstable even at room temperature and should never be used for cooking. If a pan is too hot and the oil or fat begins to smoke, it is better to discard it, clean the pan, and start over at a lower temperature.

Stir-frying is a method in which the temperature of the oil is raised to a relatively high heat, and the food is constantly moved around in the pan to avoid burning. The Chinese have perfected this method of cooking with a round bottomed pan called a wok, which ensures that only a small portion of the food is ever in contact with the hottest part of the pan at any given time. Constant agitation of the food within the pan ensures even cooking. This type of frying is generally the fastest, and in many ways is the best method to preserve the nutrients in the food. Among the best fats for stir-frying are mostly saturated fats such as lard (p. 195), which unlike peanut or canola oil, is the traditional cooking fat of China.

Deep-frying involves submerging the food completely in hot oil, and is very good to give an even distribution of heat, with very little maintenance except to remove the food before it overcooks. Deep-frying will obviously add a lot of fat to the food, some of which can be drained off in a wire mesh strainer and then padded dry with some cloth or paper towels. One problem with deep-frying is that it requires a lot of oil, which is why most people tend to use low-quality oils such as refined canola, corn, safflower and sunflower oil (see p. 67). The best oil to deep fry with are heat-stable saturated fats such as ghee (p. 194) or tallow (p. 195), but after calculating how much fat is needed even a single dish could end up being quite expensive. In traditional cultures like India where people did occasionally deep-fry their food it was only used for special occasions such as weddings, indicating just how often it should be consumed. After deep-frying the oil should be discarded, as it will have undergone some degree of thermal degradation and will continue to degrade under storage. From a health perspective deep-frying results in the production of health-damaging glycotoxins and ALEs – another good reason to limit this method of cooking to special occasions.

Sautéing is derived from the French word sauté, meaning 'to jump', referring to a similar method of frying such as stir-frying, but with a regular skillet instead of a wok. In this context however I am using the word sauté to refer to lower temperature, pan-frying methods. This method is particularly good for foods that need to cook slowly, or where time is required to get a full merging of the various flavors used during cooking. For example, finely chopped onions will burn too quickly at a high temperature, but at lower temperatures the onions can be cooked slowly and evenly to get that wonderful caramelized flavor that brings richness and flavor to a dish (note that caramelization and the Maillard reaction are unrelated). Sautéing is particularly good to tease out flavors in herbs and spices, and is usually the method undertaken when preparing Indian dishes, but is equally applicable to all types of cuisine. As the temperatures used for this method are typically low-medium to medium heat monounsaturated fats such as olive, sesame or almond oil can be safely used.

Grilling

It is hard to imagine but at one time barbeques were comparatively rare, used only on occasion during the summer months when cooking inside was too hot. Now, however, barbeques are everywhere and almost everybody has one. **Grilling** food for many people seems to be an easier and much more straightforward way to cook. Conventional thinking suggests that because grilling doesn't use any cooking fat that it somehow must be healthier. Unfortunately the small amount of fat added during cooking has less significance when compared to the inherent problems of grilling food, especially meat.

Like baking and roasting (p. 119), grilling results in Maillard reactions that lead to the production of glycotoxins, and in the case of charred meat, the formation of **heterocyclic amines (HCAs)** that have been linked to breast, colorectal and prostate cancer.[235] Additional concern comes from the production of cancer-causing compounds found in the cooking gas such as benzo(a)pyrene that are deposited on the food during grilling.[236] Charcoal grills in particular release a host of toxic compounds such as toluene, formaldehyde and acetaldehyde, as well as heavy metals including mercury and cadmium, often coating the grilled food with the residue of unburnt fuel.[237, 238, 239]

The key point to grilling safely is not to do it too often, always keep a clean cooking surface on your grill to avoid burning, and give preference to cleaner fuels such as propane gas over charcoal. Use stainless steel or cast iron grates instead of non-stick or coated ceramic cooking surfaces as these wear away and flake onto the food and become another source of contamination. Cook at a low heat and prevent the grill from flaming and charring the food. Research has shown that marinating meat before cooking as well as using herbs such as garlic helps to limit the production of heterocyclic amines.[240, 241] As a general rule of thumb, I recommend grilling no more than one to two times a week, and only on a seasonal basis.

Fermentation

Everyone likes to eat fresh food but depending on climate and season it isn't always available. Several thousand years ago our ancient ancestors discovered a unique method of food preservation that we now call **fermentation**. Unlike the heat of cooking used to break down coarse fibers that trap nutrients, fermentation makes use of micro-organisms to break down cellulose and antinutrient factors to enhance assimilation.

Apart from enhancing the bioavailability of nutrients, a key feature of fermentation is the production of an acid environment that preserves the food. This is created by the presence of **lactic acid bacteria (LAB)** including species such as *Lactobacillus, Leuconostoc, Pediococcus, Lactococcus*, and *Streptococcus*. LABs are ever-present in our environment, found on the food we eat, in our kitchens and on our bodies. The wonderful thing about preparing live-culture foods is that because these organisms are ubiquitous there are no major impediments to harnessing their benefits – they are literally free for the taking. The added benefit of eating live culture foods is that they help to replenish the gut ecology, which plays a key role in regulating immune function[242] and metabolism.[243] Fermented foods are traditionally used for bowel problems including constipation, diarrhea and gastroenteritis, and are useful for inhibiting the growth of pathogenic microbes that cause ulcers *(Helicobacter pylori)*[244] and candidiasis *(Candida albicans).*[245]

People that are new to live culture foods frequently raise concerns about botulism, a toxin that is produced by the pathogenic bacteria *Clostridium*. This concern is a hangover from canning in which preserved foods are sterilized by heat and then vacuum-sealed in a can or jar. *Clostridium* is among the least heat-sensitive of bacteria, and if the food isn't completely sterilized can survive in the canned food without ever causing noticeable spoilage. With live culture foods *Clostridium* is only one among many different naturally microorganisms and is very quickly out-competed by the lactic acid bacteria during the first stages of fermentation. If spoilage does occur and a live-culture goes bad, unlike botulism-tainted canned food, live culture foods will look, smell and taste very bad, and there will be little confusion about whether or not you should eat it.

There are a vast number of live culture foods, some of which take very little preparation and others that are a little more complex, and involve other organisms besides bacteria such as yeasts and bacterial-yeast symbionts (e.g. kefir grains). Examples of live culture foods include:

- vegetables and fruits: sauerkraut, kimchi, salsa, relish, wine, vinegar
- dairy: kefir, yogurt, cultured butter, crème fraîche, cheese
- cereal grains: sourdough bread, idli, injeera, beer, rice wine
- legumes: natto, tamari, tempeh, miso, pickled beans
- fish: fish sauce, fermented cod liver oil, ooligan grease
- meat: salami, pepperoni, blackforest ham, jinhua ham

Fermented vegetables

While many different types of food can be fermented, vegetables or 'pickles' are far and away the easiest to prepare. Most take advantage of salt or saline-rich herbs such as savory seed *(Satureja montana)* to mediate how quickly the food ferments. With less salt the food ferments quickly, while more salt tends to slow down fermentation. Examples of fermented vegetable recipes include Old-fashioned Sauerkraut (p. 159), Kimchi (p. 161) and Carrot Pickle (p. 161).

Fermented dairy

Fermented dairy products are described under the section on Dairy (p. 61), as well as in the recipes for Yogurt (p. 174) and Cultured Butter (p. 176). Another fermented dairy product is kefir, a yeast-bacterial symbiont that grows as granules, utilizing the milk sugars to turn itself into a food that resembles yogurt. While kefir is dependent upon the milk sugars for its growth, a special strain called 'water kefir' can also be used to ferment juices and sweetened teas.

Fermented cereals and legumes

Fermentation is a key step in ensuring the digestibility of foods such as cereals, legumes, nuts and seeds all of which contain antinutrient factors (ANFs) such as phytic acid and trypsin inhibitors that impair digestion and inhibit the absorption of nutrients. The procedure to ferment these foods begins with making a starter. Soak the nut, seed, grain or legume in water for 24 hours at 86°F/30°C, setting aside 10% of the soaking water after draining. The next day repeat the process with fresh ingredients, but add in the reserved soaking water. By the fourth round this results in a bacterial culture that can reduce ANFs such as the phytic acid by 96% within 24 hours of soaking.[246]

While fermentation reduces ANFs it may not remove components such as lectins,[247] and nor may the food be processed sufficiently for optimal digestion, requiring additional measures such as cooking.

Sourdough

Sourdough is a method to ferment flour made from whole cereal grains with naturally occurring yeasts and bacteria that deactivate antinutrient factors. To make a sourdough culture blend one cup of whole grain flour with one cup of chlorine-free water. Keep the starter in a warm place, such as in the kitchen, at temperatures between 70-80°F/21-26°C. After 24 hours discard half the starter and add in a half-cup flour and a half-cup purified warm water to feed the culture, and repeat again the next day. By day three this mixture will have a distinct yeasty smell, and on about day four the starter will become frothy, indicating that it is ready to use. Often a brownish alcoholic liquid ('hooch') will appear on the surface – this is normal – just mix it back into the starter. Mixing this starter with another 2-3 cups each flour and water and left to sit overnight makes a great pancake mix for the morning. To make flatbread (p. 186) mix the sourdough starter with an equal part fresh flour to make a dough, and let it rise (ferment) anywhere from 2-18 hours before baking. If you are not going to use your starter, make sure to feed it everyday by adding at least an equal volume of flour and water. Thus if you have ½ cup of starter, add at least ½ cup of flour and ½ cup water to feed it. The starter can also be stored for later use in the refrigerator, but still needs to be fed at least once a week with fresh flour and water.

Curing

For our hunter-gatherer ancestors and in traditional farming communities the availability of fresh meat and fish was seasonal, and while we now make use of freezers to preserve its quality, in the past meat was cured by drying, smoking or salting, and in a few cases, by using fermentation. **Drying** through the application of heat is the simplest method of meat preservation, and the Food and Agriculture Organization (FAO) of the United Nations has a comprehensive description of this method online (see reference).[248] While traditional methods often used low temperatures to preserve the quality and flavor of the meat, modern research indicates that if salt isn't used a temperature of at least 160°F/71°C is required to inhibit disease-causing bacteria such as *E. coli.*[249]

In relatively humid regions, such as the Pacific Northwest, traditional peoples relied upon **smoking** to preserve meat, using hardwoods such as red alder *(Alnus rubra)* and maple *(Acer macrophyllum).* The smoke from the burning wood inhibits microbial contamination and coats the meat in antioxidant resins. Unfortunately, smoke also contains cancer-causing polycyclic aromatic hydrocarbons (PAHs). The production of PAHs however is associated with hot-smoking techniques, and can be reduced significantly by using indirect, cold-smoking methods.[250]

Salting food with sea or mineral salts rich in sodium chloride is another time-honored method of food preservation, and is often used prior to drying or smoking to both flavor the meat as well as enhance preservation. A diet rich in salted foods however contributes to a high intake of sodium, which has been linked to cardiovascular disease[251] and cancer.[252] Salting food with **potassium** and **sodium nitrate/nitrite** is another method used preserve meat, and is especially useful to maintain a fresh-looking color. While both sodium and potassium nitrate occur naturally in food, the evidence suggests that the synthetic forms results in the production of chemicals called nitrosamines linked to diabetes, Alzheimer's disease, liver damage, cardiovascular disease and cancer.[253, 254] Although salted meat and fish can be acceptable dietary items, they should not be relied on excessively, better used as a food for travel or in emergencies. Salted foods should be soaked in water to remove as much salt as possible before preparation. Food containing added nitrites should be assiduously avoided.

Herbs and Spices

Herbs and spices can be added to food in a number of ways, using a medium of extraction that includes water, fat and alcohol. In herbal medicine we use all these methods to make a number of different types of extracts including teas, decoctions, medicated oils and tinctures. In cooking the methods are a little less sophisticated but are essentially the same. Herbs can be added to stocks and stews to make an herbal-food decoction, as they frequently do in Chinese cookery, or they can be fried in some kind of fat first and then added to the dish you are preparing, such as in Indian cookery. Herbs can also be extracted with alcohol in much the same way as making a tincture, letting the herbs and spices steep in alcohol for a couple weeks before straining and filtering. Herbs used as mixes (masalas), dry rubs and marinades are discussed on page 142.

The following is a list of both culinary and medicinal herbs that are suitable for use in food preparation. Each listing provides the Hindi, Chinese or other names (when indicated), the energetic properties based on flavor (p. 23), quality (p. 13) and the doshas (p. 14), as well as the basic indications for each herb. Some herbs are best prepared in soups and stews, whereas others can be used for stir-fries or fermentations. For examples of how to use these herbs, please refer to the recipe section (p. 145).

American ginseng root (xi yang shen): sweet and bitter flavor, cool and wet quality. Reduces vata and pitta. Enhances vitality, boosts immunity and nourishes the adrenals. Useful in dryness and weak lungs. Use in stocks, soups and stews, one small handful of the chopped roots per pot.

Amla fruit (Indian gooseberry): sour, sweet and astringent in flavor, cool in quality. Reduces all three doshas. Used as a general restorative and anti-aging remedy. Beneficial for indigestion, fever, hepatitis, cough, diabetes, infertility, fatigue and hemorrhage. Fresh fruit can be made into a fermented pickle with salt, much like Japanese umeboshi pickle. One small handful of the fresh dried fruit can be added to stewed fruit recipes.

Asafoetida resin (hing): pungent in flavor, warm in quality. Reduces vata and kapha. Also known as "devil's dung" due to its sulfurous odor. Used as a substitute for garlic. Enhances digestion, alleviates gas and bloating, and dispels parasites. Useful in spasmodic disorders including asthma and epilepsy. Almost all commercially prepared hing is mixed with excipients such as gum arabic or wheat flour as the pure resin is extremely potent. Hing must always be fried, either with or without oil, before eating. Use ¼ - ½ tsp of the prepared hing in stews and stir-fries. In Ayurveda, hing is most often used in the formula Hingwastak, comprised of equal parts hing, ginger, black pepper, pippali, ajwain, pink salt, cumin and black cumin (nigella). Dose is 1-2 g, twice daily, eaten with the meal as a condiment.

Ashwagandha root (withania): bitter and astringent in flavor, warm in quality. Reduces vata and kapha. Used as a general restorative to build up vitality, immunity and fertility. Has a mild sedative effect and helps to reduce anxiety. Aphrodisiac. Add 2-3 crushed dried roots to soup stock. Nepalese variety of ashwagandha is field bindweed root *(Convovulus arvensis)*.

Asparagus root (shatavari, tien men dong): sweet and bitter flavor, cool and wet quality. Reduces vata and pitta. Enhances vitality and builds the blood. Counters dryness and inflammation. Specific for women, reproductive deficiency and menopause. Aphrodisiac. Use in soups and stews, 2-3 slices of the dried root per pot.

Astragalus root (huang qi): sweet flavor, warm and dry quality. Reduces vata and kapha. Enhances vitality, boosts immunity, strengthens the lungs and promotes digestion. Useful in chronic diarrhea and excess sweating. Use in soups and stews, 5-6 slices per pot.

Basil leaf: sweet and pungent flavor, warm and dry quality. Reduces vata and kapha. Promotes appetite and digestion, alleviates gas, bloating and excess mucus. Good for cough and colds. Use ¼ cup of the fresh chopped herb as a garnish, added to soups, stews and stir-fries for the last few minutes of cooking. For the dried herb use 1 tsp to 1 tbsp, added during the initial stages of cooking, in soups, stews and stir-fries. Medicinal dose is 2-3 g, twice daily.

Bay leaf (tejpatta): pungent in flavor, warm and dry quality. Reduces vata and kapha. Promotes digestion, alleviates gas and bloating, dispels excess mucus. Use 2-3 bay leaves in stocks, soups, stews and fermented vegetables.

Black Mustard seed (kalirai, sarson): pungent and bitter in flavor, warming in quality. Reduces vata and kapha. Stimulates digestion, promotes circulation and dispels mucus. Use about 1-2 tsp, fried in butter or ghee as part of an Indian masala. Good quality seeds are small and bright purple in color.

Black Pepper fruit (gulki, hu jiao): pungent in flavor, warming in quality. Reduces vata and kapha. Stimulates and promotes good digestion and circulation; dispels mucus. Use ½ - 1 tsp in most dishes. While whole peppercorns can be added to soups and stews, fresh-cracked pepper should be added towards the end of cooking.

Calendula flower: bitter and astringent in flavor, cooling in quality. Reduces pitta and kapha. Promotes wound-healing, reduces inflammation and supports the liver. Imparts a cheery yellow pigment to soups and stews. Add a handful to soups.

Caraway seed: pungent and bitter in flavor, warming in quality. Reduces vata and kapha. Traditional herb of northern Europe with a strong flavor that combines well with garlic. Enhances digestion and alleviates colic and gas. Use ½ - 1 tsp in stir-fries, stews, fermented vegetables and flatbreads.

Cardamom seed, black (badi elachi, xiang dou kou): pungent and bitter in flavor, cool and dry in quality. Reduces pitta and kapha. Useful for nausea, indigestion and excess mucus. Stated to have sedative and anti-toxic properties. Black cardamom is often dried over a fire and has a darker, smokier flavor than the green cardamom. Use 3-5 pods in stews.

Cardamom seed, green (choti elachi): sweet and pungent in flavor, cool and dry in quality. Reduces kapha. Useful for nausea, indigestion, colic, excess mucus, cough, dyspnea, urinary problems and hemorrhoids. Green cardamom is an infertile hybrid with a much more delicate flavor than black cardamom, making it suitable for desserts, as well as stews and grain dishes. Often mixed with coffee to ameliorate the negative effects of caffeine. Use 10-15 of the fresh cracked pods in stews, stir-fries, stewed fruits and confections.

Chickweed: bitter in flavor, cool and dry in quality. Reduces all three doshas. Useful for general nutrition as well as to reduce inflammation and to promote wound healing. Useful for acne, eczema, liver problems, lipoma and gout. Use fresh as a potherb, one bunch chopped into salads, soups and stews.

Chili fruit (mirch, la jiao): pungent in flavor, warm and dry in quality. Reduces kapha. Dispels mucus, enhances appetite, promotes circulation and stimulates the mind and senses. Heat sensation depends on the variety of chili, and can range from mild (e.g. paprika), moderate (e.g. cayenne) to exceptionally hot (e.g. habañero). Flavor and pungency is reduced with roasting, smoking and cooking. Use ¼ tsp to 1 tsp in stews and stir-fries, depending on what stage during cooking the chili is added.

Chinese Angelica root (dang gui): sweet, pungent and bitter flavor, warm and wet quality. Reduces vata. Enhances vitality, builds the blood, dispels coldness, promotes circulation, relieves pain and lubricates the body. Indicated in female reproductive deficiency and menopause. Has a strong celery-like flavor similar to lovage. Use a small handful of the sliced root in stocks and soups.

Chinese Ginseng root (ren shen): sweet, pungent and bitter flavor, warm in quality. Reduces vata and kapha. Enhances vitality and invigorates, warms the body, promotes circulation, lowers blood sugar and builds stamina and strength. Aphrodisiac. **Red ginseng** is a lesser quality steam-treated ginseng, which preserves the herb and gives it a red color, said to impart a more warming quality. There are a huge number of varieties and grades of Chinese ginseng, the largest and heaviest commanding the greatest price. Small ginseng rootlets however are actually still very potent, and can be obtained at a fraction of the cost. Use a handful of rootlets in soups, stews and confections.

Chinese red dates (hong zao): sweet flavor, warm and wet in quality. Reduces vata and pitta. Enhances vitality and boosts immunity. Calms the mind, balances and restores the nervous system. Best are fresh dates. Remove seeds and use 1-2 handfuls in soups and stews.

Chinese yam rhizome (shan yao): sweet flavor, cool and wet quality. Reduces vata and pitta. Restores and energizes digestion, strengthens lungs and boosts immunity. Fresh is used as a medicinal food in relatively large amounts, often in traditional confections. Dried is used in smaller amounts in stocks, soups and stews. Use to make stock or soup, 1-2 small handfuls per pot.

Cinnamon bark (dalchini, rou gui): sweet and pungent flavor, warm and dry quality. Reduces vata and kapha. Promotes circulation and enhances vitality. Helps stop bleeding and diarrhea, lowers blood sugar. Use 2-3 sticks, or a small handful of the broken bark in stocks, soups, stews, stewed fruit and confections.

Clove flower (lavang): pungent, bitter and sweet flavor, cold and dry quality. Reduces kapha and pitta. Promotes digestion, dispels colic, reduces pain and inflammation. One clove can be chewed to treat dental pain, improve breath and decrease mucus. Use 8-10 cloves in soups, stews and grain dishes.

Codonopsis root (dang shen): sweet flavor, warm and wet in quality. Reduces vata and kapha. Enhances vitality, dispels fatigue, strengthens lungs and boosts digestion. Also known as "poor man's ginseng". Use 4-5 roots per pot in soups and stews.

Coriander seed (dhaniya): pungent and bitter in flavor, cool and dry in quality. Reduces pitta and kapha. Both seeds ("coriander") and tender greens ("cilantro") are used. Decreases inflammation and promotes detoxification, reputedly useful for heavy metal toxicity. Useful in gas, colic and fever. Use 1-2 tbsp of the fresh powdered seed in soups and stews, and a half-bunch of the fresh chopped herb as a garnish.

Cumin seed (jeera): pungent and bitter in flavor, warm and dry in quality. Reduces vata and kapha. Useful in indigestion, colic, gas and bloating. Used in premenstrual syndrome, during pregnancy to alleviate nausea and with breastfeeding to promote lactation. **Black cumin (kalonji, nigella)** is a similar species with a similar flavor, quality and use. Use 1 tsp to 1 tbsp in soups, stews, stir-fries, grain dishes and fermented vegetables.

Curry leaf (karipatti): pungent and bitter in flavor, warm in quality. Reduces all three doshas. Used to stimulate appetite and promote digestion. Highly aromatic, provides a distinct flavor to Indian dishes, and is the origin of the English word 'curry'. Prefer fresh over dried, 1-2 sprigs separated from stem, stir-fried in fat and added to soups, stews and stir-fries near the end of cooking.

Dandelion (dudal, pu gong ying): bitter in flavor, cool and dry in quality. Reduces pitta and kapha. Fresh herb is used as a salad green and potherb, dried herb used as a potassium-sparing diuretic in bladder infection, kidney stones, hypertension and edema. Root is used to stimulate flow of bile, useful in gallstones, constipation and PMS. Use the fresh leaf in salads and soups. Dried root can be roasted and ground into a powder, and used as a substitute for coffee.

Dill seed, herb (sowa): pungent and bitter, warm and dry in quality. Reduces vata and kapha. Used to alleviate nausea, gas and bloating, constipation and cough. Good for infant colic. Seed can be added to fermented foods, soups, stews and grain dishes. Use ½-1 tsp. The fresh herb has a milder property, and a small handful can be chopped and added to food as a garnish.

Epazote: pungent in taste, warm and dry in quality. Reduces vata and kapha. Used to treat indigestion, colic, cough and congestion, PMS and intestinal parasites. Frequently used in legume dishes to counteract flatulence. Use no more than about ¼ cup of the finely chopped fresh herb, or 1 tsp of the dried leaf.

Fennel seed, herb (sonf, hui xiang): pungent and bitter, warm and light in quality. Reduces vata and kapha. Used to alleviate weak appetite, indigestion, colic and fever, gas and bloating. Promotes breastmilk, useful for infant colic. Use 1-2 tsp of the seed in fermented foods, soups, stews and grain dishes. Both the fresh and dried leaves have a milder property, added to food as a garnish. The fresh rootstock can be added to salads, soups, stews and fermentations.

Fenugreek seed, herb (methi): bitter and sweet, warm in quality. Reduces vata and kapha. Used to stimulate the appetite and raise the natural fire of the body, making it useful for digestive problems including constipation, colic, parasites and hemorrhoids. Also used to dispel fatigue, strengthen the heart and balance blood sugar. One small handful of the fresh leaf can be added as a garnish near the end of cooking. Use ½ - 1 tsp of the seed in stews.

Garlic bulb (lashun, da suan): all flavors except sour, warm and wet in quality. Reduces vata and kapha. Raw garlic is pungent and stimulating, dispels mucus, infection and parasites. Cooked garlic is nourishing, strengthening and fertility-promoting. Aphrodisiac. Use raw in fermented foods, or mix with fatty foods such as avocado or olive oil, 1-2 cloves per serving, up to an entire head per dish. Add to soups, stews, stir-fries or roast in the oven.

Ginger rhizome (sonth): pungent in flavor, warm and light in quality. Reduces vata and kapha. Stimulates digestion and circulation, used in excess mucus, nausea, cough, joint pain, headache and edema. Use ¼ - 1 tsp of the fresh ground powder in soups and stews. **Fresh ginger (adrak, sheng jiang)** is similar but comparatively mild and not so drying and heating, used for indigestion, nausea, colds, flu and fever. Chop one thumb-sized piece and add to soups, stews and stir-fries.

Goji fruit (gou zi, wolfberry): sweet in flavor, cool and wet in quality. Reduces vata and pitta. Enhances vitality, builds the blood and nourishes the liver, eyes and lungs. Use about ¼ cup in soups, stews and grain dishes.

Gotu kola (brahmi, ji xue cao): bitter in flavor, cool and dry in quality. Reduces all three doshas. Antiinflammatory herb with wound-healing properties, useful in nervous disorders, stress and exhaustion. Indicated in skin conditions including acne and eczema, as well as dementia, poor memory and concentration problems. Use a few leaves as a salad green or pot herb.

Hemp seed (huo ma ren): sweet in flavor, warm and wet in quality. Reduces vata. Rich in protein, omega 3 fats and fiber. Whole seed used to lubricate bowels and gently stimulate bowel movements in chronic or occasional constipation. Nourishing and restorative, reduces inflammation. Use 1-2 tbsp of the freshly hulled 'hearts' sprinkled over food or as a snack. Cooking destroys benefits.

Holy Basil leaf (tulsi): pungent and bitter, warm in quality. Reduces vata and kapha. Used in weak digestion, cough, hepatitis and skin disease. Stimulates mind and senses, benefits the heart. Use 1 tsp of the fresh dried leaves in soups and stews.

Juniper fruit (ahrahr): sweet, pungent and bitter in flavor, warm in quality. Reduces vata and kapha. General nutritive that stimulates and purifies the blood, indicated in skin disease, arthritis and rheumatism. Specific to urinary tract infection. Stimulates digestion of heavy foods like meat, adding a sweet coniferous flavor. Use one handful in soups, stews, and stewed fruits.

Lemonbalm leaf: pungent and bitter in flavor, cool in quality. Reduces all three doshas. Stimulates digestion, dispels mucus, reduces inflammation and fever. Calms the mind, benefits the heart and circulation. Use 1 tsp - 1 tbsp in soups and stews to add a citrus flavor.

Licorice (yashti, gan cao): sweet, pungent and bitter in flavor, cool and wet in quality. Reduces vata and pitta. Reduces heat and inflammation, counters dryness and irritation. Helps to counter exhaustion, stress and deficiency states. Useful in gastric reflux, ulcers, cough, urinary tract infection and adrenal deficiency. Use 2-3 crushed roots in soups and stews, 1 tsp in boiled milk.

Lily bulb (bai he): sweet and bitter in flavor, cool in quality. Reduces vata and pitta. Moistens and nourishes the respiratory system in dry cough and sore throat. Calms and balances the mind, helps with recuperation after a fever or chronic illness. Use one small handful of the dried roots in stocks, soups and stews.

Long Pepper fruit (pippali, pipal): pungent and sweet in flavor, warm in quality. Reduces vata and kapha. Used for indigestion, colds, cough, fever, asthma, poor circulation, diabetes and skin disease. Rejuvenating and aphrodisiac. Use ½ - 1 tsp of the fresh ground fruit in stir-fries, stewed fruit and confections, or as a garnish in soups and stews.

Marjoram leaf: pungent and bitter, warm in quality. Reduces vata and kapha. A cultivated variety of oregano, with milder flavor and taste. Indicated for indigestion, colds, cough and poor circulation. Use 1 tsp of the dried herb in soups, stews and stir-fries.

Mint leaf (pudina, bo he): pungent and bitter in flavor, warm in quality. Reduces vata and kapha. Refers to a large variety of related plants, from the sweet and mild Spearmint *(Mentha spicata)* to the rather pungent Field Mint (Bo He, *Mentha arvensis)* and Peppermint *(Mentha piperita)*. Used for indigestion, colic, fever, cough, headache and skin disease. Use a handful of the chopped fresh leaves in fermented foods or as a garnish for soups, stews and grain dishes. For the dried herb, use 1-2 tsp in the latter stages of cooking for soups, stews and stewed fruit. Loses its aroma with over-cooking.

Nettle leaf: bitter and astringent in flavor, cool in quality. Reduces all three doshas. High in minerals, and a natural restorative to the bones, skin, hair and nails. Purifies and alkalizes the blood, clears up skin issues, reduces the pain of arthritis and gout. Use 1-2 tbsp of the dried herb in stocks, soups and stews. The fresh green young nettle harvested in springtime can be eaten as a vegetable.

Nutmeg fruit (jaiphal): sweet, pungent and bitter in flavor, warm in quality. Reduces vata and kapha. Used for bad breath, indigestion, colic and diarrhea. Alleviates congestion and cough.

A reputed aphrodisiac, nutmeg reduces pain and benefits insomnia. Use ¼ - ½ tsp of the fresh grated seed in stews, stewed fruits, boiled milk and confections.

Orange peel (chen pi): sweet, pungent and bitter in flavor, warm in quality. Reduces vata and kapha. Dried peel enhances digestion and absorption, reduces nausea, gas, bloating and excess mucus. Chinese variety chen pi is dried tangerine peel. Use a small handful in soups, stews and stewed fruit to provide a citrus flavor.

Oregano leaf: pungent and bitter in flavor, warm in quality. Reduces vata and kapha. Enhances digestion, inhibits infection, dispels mucus and promotes circulation. Use fresh herb as a garnish, in stir-fries and in fermented vegetables. Dried herb is used in amounts of 1-2 tsp in soups and stews.

Parsley leaf: pungent and bitter in flavor, warm in quality. Reduces vata and kapha. Freshens breath, enhances digestion and purifies the blood. Fresh parsley is preferred. Used in fermented vegetable dishes and salads, and as a garnish for soups, stews and grain dishes. Of the dried herb, use 1-2 tbsp in soups, stews and grain dishes.

Peony root (bai shao): bitter and sour in flavor, cool in quality. Reduces vata and pitta. Enhances vitality and nourishes blood, reduces spasm and pain. Useful in PMS, menopause, cough, asthma, and liver problems. Use 3-5 slices per pot in soups and stews.

Pink salt (sanchal): salty and pungent in flavor, cool and wet in quality. Reduces all three doshas. Enhances digestion, benefits eyes, restores electrolytes, nourishes and rejuvenates. Use as a substitute for regular sea salt. Has a mild garlicky flavor due to high sulfur content.

Polygonum root (he shou wu): bitter, sweet, and astringent in flavor, warm in quality. Reduces vata and pitta. Rejuvenating herb used in the treatment of aging. Lubricates and nourishes the blood, skin, hair and intestines. Useful for anemia, dizziness, anxiety, blurred vision, infertility and weak joints. Use one handful of the sliced dried root per pot to make soup stock.

Poria fungus (fu ling): sweet in flavor, warm and dry in quality. Reduces vata and kapha. Traditionally used to strengthen digestion, dispel mucus and drain edema. Also used as a general nutritive to promote growth and prevent aging. Promotes relaxation and benefits insomnia. Use 1-2 small handfuls of the dried sliced fungus when making soup stock.

Prickly Ash berry (tejphal, hua jiao): pungent and bitter in flavor, hot and dry in quality. Reduces vata and kapha. Used to enhance digestion, promote circulation, reduce mucus, kill parasites, and stimulate the spleen and immunity. When chewed promotes salivation and relieves gum pain. Also known as **Szechuan pepper.** Used 1-2 tsp of the crushed fruit in stir-fries, soups and stews.

Rehmannia root, cured (shu di huang): sweet in flavor, warm and wet in quality. Reduces vata and pitta. Enhances vitality and builds the blood. Useful in anemia, infertility, PMS and menopause. Anti-aging remedy for both sexes. Use one handful per pot when making soup stock.

Rose blossom (gulab, mei gui ha): bitter, astringent and sweet in flavor, cool and dry in quality. Reduces all three doshas. Cools and dehydrates the body, calms and pacifies the nervous system, benefits the heart. Reduces fever and inflammation, stops bleeding and tones the skin and mucus membranes. Useful in PMS. Use in sweets, syrups and confections, as well as in fermented beverages and fortified wines.

Rosemary leaf: pungent and bitter in flavor, warm and dry in quality. Reduces vata and kapha. Opens and clears the channels, reduces mucus, and enhances digestion. Boosts mood, concentration and enhances circulation. Use fresh or dried whole leaves, 1-2 tbsp in soups, stews and stir-fries.

Sage leaf: bitter and pungent in flavor, cool and dry in quality. Reduces kapha and pitta. Enhances digestion, reduces inflammation and inhibits infection. Reduces mucus and opens the airways. Reduces fever and sweating. Use 1-2 tsp of the crushed dried herb in soups, stews and stir-fries.

Sea salt: salty in flavor, warm and dry in quality. Reduces vata. Promotes appetite and enhances digestion. Used to restore electrolytes, liquefy mucus and balance the nervous system. Sea salt is warm in quality while pink salt (sanchal) is cooling. Also used to help ferment food (p. 124). Both sea salt and pink salt have a balanced ratio of sodium to other trace minerals, whereas table salt is pure sodium chloride mixed with anticaking agents such as sodium ferrocyanide as well as inorganic iodine. Use up to 1 tsp of sea salt or pink salt in recipes, or ¼ - ½ tsp per serving.

Seaweed: salty in flavor, warm in quality. Reduces vata and kapha. Refers to a huge variety of species that vary in flavor and consistency including dulse, bladderwrack, kelp, wakame, hijiki, arame, laver, kombu and sea lettuce. All seaweeds are an excellent natural source of macrominerals and trace minerals. Useful for nourishment, detoxification, and to promote circulation. Boosts metabolism and enhances thyroid function. Use about 10 - 25 grams in stocks, soups and stews.

Slippery Elm: sweet in flavor, cold in quality. Reduces vata and pitta. Inner bark is a useful demulcent herb to soothe inflammation and dryness. Useful in dry cough, heartburn, ulcers, and intestinal inflammation. Prepare as a porridge, or cook in boiled milk, 1 tbsp per cup.

Solomon's seal root (yu zhu): sweet in flavor, cold in quality. Reduces vata and pitta. Nourishing and soothing, useful in deficiency states with inflammation. Indicated in dry cough, thirst, weight loss and constipation. Use a small handful of the dried, sliced root in stocks and soups.

Tamarind fruit (imli): sour in flavor, warm in quality. Reduces all three doshas. Enhances appetite and stimulates digestion. Dispels mucus, infection and colds. Useful for exhaustion, dizziness, thirst, and mental fatigue. Supports the liver and the heart. For the dried fruit, soak a lemon-sized piece in hot water for 15 minutes, and then squeeze out and strain the juice. For tamarind paste use 1 tbsp mixed with a little hot water, and add to soups and curries. Tamarind bestows a delightful tangy flavor.

Tarragon leaf: bitter and pungent in flavor, hot and dry in quality. Reduces vata and kapha. Used in colds and flu, stimulates digestion, kills parasites and promotes menstruation. When fresh, use the leaves stripped from one sprig, or 1 tsp of the dried herb, in soups, stews and fermented vegetables.

Thyme leaf: bitter and pungent in flavor, hot and dry in quality. Reduces pitta and kapha. Used in colds, cough and flu, and to stimulate digestion and circulation. Use fresh, the leaves stripped from 3-5 sprigs, or 1-2 tsp of the freshly dried herb in soups and stews.

Turmeric rhizome (haldi, jiang huang): bitter and pungent in flavor, hot and dry in quality. Reduces kapha and pitta. Used to promote liver health, skin complexion, balance blood sugar, inhibit infection, kill parasites and reduce inflammation. Effective as a gargle with salt water for sore throats, and boiled in milk to alleviate cough. Believed to have mild contraceptive effects. Good quality powder is bright orange with pungent, aromatic flavor. Add ½ - 1 tsp to stir-fries and stews – too much will ruin the flavor of the dish.

Wild Celery seed (ajwain): bitter and pungent in flavor, hot and dry in quality. Reduces vata and kapha. Useful in sore throat, colds and flu, indigestion, colic, bloating and gas. Promotes good circulation and alleviates joint pain. Used in pregnancy for morning sickness and to promote milk while breastfeeding. Use ½ - 1 tsp in stocks, soups, stews and fermented vegetables.

Masalas, Rubs and Marinades

There are a number of ways to instill flavor and the medicinal qualities of herbs and spices into the food we eat, and here I have divided them into masalas (mixtures), rubs and marinades. A **masala** is just a spice mixture used in Indian cooking, and is really no different in essence from a Mexican mole or French Herbs de Provence – it simply refers to a combination of flavors. In Indian cuisine a masala forms the character of a dish, particularly in soups, stir-fries and stews. Typically the masala is either dry roasted or fried in fat for a few minutes before the other foods are added, to render the flavor and medicinal properties of the herbs and spices.

Although masala is an Indian word, I suggest it be adopted into the English language as a concept whose time has come. Behind its meaning as a spice mixture, masala refers to a diverse tapestry of experience, juxtaposed and yet harmonious, reflecting not just our own unique features as individuals but the diversity found in food, culture, society and life. As a concept the word masala teaches us that both flavor and medicine are intensely personal experiences, and as the Arabic saying goes, there are as many paths to God as there are rays of the sun. Nonetheless, just as people group together so do flavors and hence each culture has a distinctive theme for its masala. When I cook I think along these themes to create my own unique voice within this tapestry of taste.

What follows are flavor combinations along several different themes. Experiment and play with these flavors, using different amounts of each type of herb or flavor, using only some or all, and adding others I haven't listed. Use a little and the flavor is subtle – use a lot and you get a big taste. Herbs with an asterisk (*) are those you might want to use in smaller proportions compared to the others due to their dominant flavor. Many of the recipes in this book utilize these flavor themes, and so check out the recipe section (p. 145) to see how to use these flavors in action.

Theme	Herbs and flavors
French/English	thyme, savory, tarragon, marjoram, fennel, leek, chervil, parsley, sage*, salt
Mediterranean	garlic, basil, rosemary, oregano, black pepper, bay leaf*, salt
Eastern European	caraway, dill, rosemary, garlic, paprika, bay leaf*, salt
Persian	leek, parsley, basil, mint, garlic, coriander, fenugreek*, cumin*, salt
Indian (savory)	cumin, black mustard, coriander, ginger, curry leaf, turmeric*, ajwain*, fenugreek*, hing*, pink salt*
Indian (sweet)	cumin, coriander, cardamom, cinnamon, black pepper, ginger, clove*, nutmeg*, saffron*, salt
Thai	ginger, Thai basil, garlic, soy sauce, lemongrass*, galangal*, fish sauce*, red chili, coconut or peanut
Chinese (savory)	black bean (douchi), garlic, ginger, sesame oil, soy sauce, fish sauce
Chinese (sweet)	star anise, ginger, Szechuan pepper*, cinnamon, clove*, soy sauce, garlic, cilantro
Japanese	tamari, miso, ginger, shisho, seaweed, sesame seed, rice vinegar, umeboshi*
Pacific Northwest	juniper, hazelnut, nettle, sea asparagus (Salicornia spp.), wild onion, wild mint, wild celery (Lomatium spp.)
Mexican	dried or smoked chili (e.g. chipotle), garlic, oregano, basil, cinnamon, cumin, coriander/cilantro, epazote, nutmeg*

A **dry rub** is a dry masala that is used to flavor a piece of meat for roasting or grilling, whereas a **wet rub** or **paste** is a masala mixed with a little liquid, such as oil, wine or fruit juice. To make a rub, finely grind the herbs and spices and then vigorously massage and rub the masala into the piece of meat. A masala can also be used as a rub for baked and grilled vegetables as well, with our without a little oil or fat.

A **marinade** is a masala blended with an acid solution like wine, beer, lime juice, pineapple juice or vinegar. The acids help to tenderize the meat and allow for the flavors to penetrate. Marinades are prepared fresh, and then applied to the meat, ensuring that every part is bathed in flavor. The meat is allowed to sit in the marinade for several hours (2-8 hours) or overnight in the fridge before cooking. Marinades are particularly good for stir-fried, grilled and baked dishes. Marinades are also used for some vegetarian dishes as well, such as grilled vegetables, baked vegetables and tofu.

Section Three: Medicinal Recipes

Stocks and Soups

Soup Stock

Knowing how to make soup stock is a basic requirement of cooking, but most people aren't aware that making soup is a metaphor for the activities of digestion. Digestive issues are so common nowadays, and most people so confused on the subject, that it's good to get back to basics. If the digestion is like a fire, all the care needed to properly restore digestion is understood by the same knowledge it takes to build and maintain a fire. And if you have ever built a fire, then you know that there is more to it than just holding a match to a log. You know that you need to 'enkindle' the fire, using light, easily combustible materials such as paper and thin strips of wood such as cedar kindling. Only once you have a little fire going can you thrown on a big log.

The digestive fire is best enkindled by light, easily digestible foods, and for this purpose there is no better food than soup. To make such a soup, we need to have some base ingredients, and these can include anything and everything from vegetable trimmings and peelings, to any kind of animal bones or carcass. Simply throw all these ingredients into a pot, cover with water, and let simmer for 12-24 hrs. Especially for stocks containing animal fats, make sure to avoid bringing the stock to a boil as this will cause the fats to peroxidize and produce undesirable off-flavors.

Most frequently I use soups as a medium to build and restore the skeletal system, using ingredients such as chicken or turkey bones, lamb bones and beef marrowbones. These bones contain valuable nutrients such as calcium, phosphorous, magnesium, glucosamine and chondroitin that our bodies can use to build and enhance bone health, to prevent and treat osteoporosis and arthritis. To render these constituents bioavailable, add in a little vinegar to create a slightly acid medium that will pull these minerals into the broth. To spike up the nutrient profile of these bone soups, I frequently recommend adding in seaweed such as kelp or dulse. Sea vegetables are truly one of nature's super foods, not only as the single most abundant source of minerals compared to any land-based food, but also to boost metabolism and promote detoxification. In addition, there are any number of medicinal plants that can be added to boost the healing properties of the soup.

Ingredients
3-5 lbs of bones
2-3 handfuls of seaweed
vegetable trimmings and peels
2 tbsp apple cider vinegar

Directions
    Place ingredients into a large stockpot and fill to the top with water. Heat on high until almost boiling, then reduce to a simmer and let cook for 12-24 hours. *Do not boil.* When done, strain and then store in the refrigerator. When cool, the fat will rise to the top and can be skimmed off. When preparing soup with marrowbones however, as well as in people suffering from immunodeficiency or excessive dryness (vata dosha), the fattiness of the stock can be retained as a medicinal ingredient. I frequently recommend bone broths to perimenopausal women to maintain bone density, and include herbs such as shatavari, peony, dang gui, rehmannia and nettle.

Medicinal Mushroom Broth

    A mushroom broth is in many respects the closest we can come to a nourishing bone broth without using animal products, but it is also quite distinct and very unique. The Chinese have a particularly evolved use of mushroom broths, not just for flavor, but as medicinal foods. The basic Chinese mushroom broth is made with dried Chinese brown mushrooms, i.e. dried shiitake mushrooms. Shiitake mushroom is used as a general restorative in Chinese medicine, and has been shown to have a number of medicinal benefits, demonstrating antitumor, immune-regulating, liver-supportive and antimicrobial effects.[255]

Ingredients
2-3 oz dried Chinese brown mushrooms
1-2 quarts water

Rinse the dried mushrooms in a colander, and soak for 20 minutes in cool water. Drain, and put mushrooms in a pot with fresh water, bring to a boil, and simmer for one hour. Strain broth through a colander, and squeeze out any remaining moisture in the mushrooms, and compost. The broth is now ready for use in soups and stews.

To boost the mineral content, add in any vegetable peelings or ends, such as carrot tops, broccoli stems etc. in the soup to boost mineral content. If you feel like you're getting a cold or flu, use the mushroom stock as a base and cook sliced ginger, garlic and the whites of several green onions for 10 minutes, and garnish with green onion. Seaweeds such as kelp or dulse can be added as well to boost mineral content, detoxify the body and enhance metabolism. Herbs such as astragalus, American ginseng and shatavari can be added to boost immunity and support the adrenals. The Chinese fungus fu ling can also be added, to enhance the nourishing properties of the stock and remove excess fluid (edema) from the body. Western herbs such as nettle and oatstraw can be added to nourish the skin and hair.

Mulligatawny Soup

Mulligatawny is derived from the Tamil word 'milagutanni', 'milagu' referring to pepper and 'tanni' referring to water. Mulligatawny then is a kind of pepper water, used to enhance digestion and treat colds and flu. Traditionally this was made as a soup, whether using vegetable or meat stock. As the intent with Mulligatawny Soup is to enhance digestion and clear phlegm (kapha), only a stock that has had the fat skimmed from it should be used. Heavy, greasy foods are typically contraindicated in weak digestion.

Ingredients
2 cups soup stock
1 tsp cumin seed
½ tsp black mustard seed
1 tsp coriander seed powder
½ tsp black pepper
½ tsp turmeric powder
½ tsp salt

Chopped fresh cilantro or green onion to taste

Directions

Put stock in a pot and warm until hot. In a separate pan, dry roast the cumin and black mustard seed at medium heat until the mustard begins to pop. Add in the coriander, pepper, turmeric and salt, and roast for another 30 seconds. Add this mixture into the soup, and garnish with cilantro or green onion.

This soup can also be used as a base for more complex recipes. Add a little cooked rice, roasted urad dhal or finely shredded chicken to enhance strength and build energy once digestion improves.

Garden Vegetable Soup

This recipe is based on a favorite that my Grandmother used to make. Delicately flavored with common vegetables and herbs this soup is the perfect mid-day meal or appetizer. With its mild flavor this soup has a balancing, harmonizing action, helping to rehydrate the tissues and restore electrolytes. From an Ayurvedic perspective this soup balances all three doshas, and helps to dispel toxins (ama), and is a good food during any kind of detoxification regimen (see p. 219).

Ingredients
4 cups soup stock
1 onion, finely chopped
2 stalks celery, finely chopped
1 carrot, diced
2 cloves garlic, minced
1 tsp dried parsley
1 tsp savory
1 tsp marjoram
1 tsp thyme
1 tbsp olive oil
salt and pepper to taste

<u>Directions</u>

In a medium sized pot sauté all the ingredients, including the herbs, at medium heat, just until the onions become translucent. Add stock, increase heat just until the stock begins to bubble then turn down and simmer for 10-20 minutes. Add salt and pepper to taste.

This basic vegetable soup has countless variations, depending on the vegetables and herbs. To give a more Asian flavor, use herbs such as ginger, garlic, chives, tamari and a dash of toasted sesame oil. For a Mexican flavor add in tomatoes, cayenne, oregano, garlic and fresh cilantro. You might also consider using wild plants such as nettles and lambsquarters that might be popping up in your backyard.

This soup is a good base for other dishes, and can be poured over well-cooked grains such as rice, barley or buckwheat to make a soupier version of the Breakfast Bowl (p. 182).

Borscht

Borscht is an important dish of both central Asia and Eastern Europe, eaten from Azerbaijan in the Caucasus Mountains all the way up through the Ukraine to Lithuania in northern Europe. Although prepared with a number of ingredients including cabbage and garlic, the nutritive and healing properties of borscht are a testament to beet root *(Beta vulgaris)*, a reddish-purple colored root that is loaded with antioxidants including betanin, vulgaxanthin, lutein and zeaxanthin. Studies have shown that beet root supports liver detoxification,[256] enhances life expectancy in prostate cancer,[257] and lowers blood pressure, protects the arteries and decreases platelet aggregation in cardiovascular disease.[258] The sweet, grounding taste of beets is excellent for reducing both vata and pitta, useful in supporting the liver and bowels to promote regularity. Beets are also a good way to track intestinal transit time, to see how quickly the food is moving through your gut. While it is normal for beets to color the feces and urine after eating, high levels of beet root pigments in the urine (beeturia) can be an indication of low stomach acid, anemia, malabsorption syndrome or food allergies.[259]

Borscht is traditionally made with lacto-fermented beets (see p. 126), although because the dish is cooked it cannot be considered to be a probiotic food. To make soured beets scrub well and cut off the ends. Grate the beets and add 3 tbsp (45 mL) salt per five pounds (2.2 kg) of beet. Mix well in a large bowl and then stuff inside a crock or mason jar and let sit between 1 – 4 weeks to ferment, making sure the brine that forms rises above the surface of the beets to avoid spoilage. Once ready, the beets can be incorporated into the recipe below, omitting the red wine vinegar.

Ingredients
2 cups grated beet root
1 small red cabbage, grated
2 carrots, grated
2 stalks celery, finely chopped
2 red onions, finely chopped
3-4 cloves garlic, minced
1 tsp caraway seed
2 bay leaves
2 tbsp red wine vinegar (if not using soured beets)
4-5 cups soup stock
2-3 tbsp butter

Directions
   In a large pot sauté the onion, garlic and celery in butter until translucent, and add in the caraway and bay leaves. Add in the grated beets, carrot and cabbage, and continue to sauté for 10-15 minutes, until the vegetables are soft. If not using soured beets, add in the red wine vinegar and cook for another few minutes, and then add in the soup stock. Bring to a boil, reduce to a simmer and cook for several hours. Serve with a dollop of sour cream (p. 176) and chives, and serve with flatbread (p. 186).

Vegetable Dishes

Greek Salad

Greek salad is a particularly popular food in the summertime when it's hot and cooked food is just too warming. The combination of the watery cucumbers, the salty feta and the tangy vinegar all help to restore electrolytes on a hot day.

<u>Ingredients</u>
2 cucumbers, chopped
2 tomatoes, chopped
¼ sweet red onion, finely sliced
¼ cup goat feta cheese, crumbled
2-3 tbsp olive oil
2-3 tbsp live-culture red wine vinegar
1 tsp fresh cracked black pepper
2-3 tbsp fresh oregano (finely chopped), or 1 tsp dried oregano (freshly rubbed)

<u>Directions</u>
Chop up the vegetables and add them to the salad bowl. Add the feta cheese, olive oil, vinegar, black pepper and chopped fresh oregano. If you are using dried oregano make sure to rub it with your palms a bit to break it down and release the essential oils. For variation, add in chopped parsley or kalamata olives. To make it more of a meal add in avocados, or mix with freshly cooked grains such as quinoa.

Chinese Greens and Arame

Greens are an important food to include at every meal, supplying valuable minerals, phytochemicals and fiber, as well as supporting the liver and bowels to promote detoxification. Chinese cookery is notable for its great diversity of cooking greens, from the cruciferous greens such as bok choy, sui choy, choy sum and gai lan, to other species including amaranth greens (hin choy) and spinach (san choy). Beyond these, any number of greens can substituted for this recipe, such as mustard greens, turnip greens, cabbage, kale, rapini, chard and beet greens. All the greens have slightly different cooking times, the more delicate ones cooking more quickly, and the denser, more fibrous greens taking a little longer. Arame is a type of seaweed that has a mild taste and is easy to cook with, and as a super food, adds to the overall healing potential of this dish.

Ingredients
2 oz arame
1 lb baby bok choy, ends trimmed off
3-4 cloves garlic, crushed
1 tbsp salted Chinese black beans (douchi)
1 thumb-sized piece of ginger
2 tbsp extra virgin sesame oil and/or pork fat
1 tbsp tamari
½ tsp fish sauce

Directions
Soak arame in room temperature water for 10-15 minutes, and then drain. In a pan at medium heat, add oil, crushed garlic, ginger, black beans and arame and stir. After a minute, add in the greens, stirring frequently. As the greens reduce in volume and become bright green, add in the fish sauce and tamari. Continue stir-frying for another half minute or so, and then you're done. Serves 2-4 people.

This basic Chinese stir-fry recipe has endless variations. Need to boost the immune system? Throw in some chopped Shiitake mushrooms with the arame. Want a quick high-protein meal? Slice up a block of organic soft tofu, and add it just before the tamari and fish sauce, stirring gently. Instead of tofu, throw in some broken almonds or cashews with the arame. You might even experiment with stronger tasting seaweeds such as hijiki, kelp or dulse (just remember to soak them for at least an hour). Use your imagination!

Spicy Saag

Saag refers to any kind of stir-fried greens in Indian cookery, prepared with the characteristic Indian spices such as cumin and black mustard seed. While spinach is most commonly used nowadays, saag can be made with any kind of greens, such as amaranth greens found in Chinese markets as hin choy and Indian markets as chaulai. I frequently use the kale and chard in my garden. To boost the nutrient content, I also add in other herbs such as fresh cilantro and fenugreek (methi), or use curry leaf instead.

Ingredients
1-2 lbs of amaranth greens, chopped into 1 inch chunks
½ bunch finely chopped fenugreek (methi)
½ bunch finely chopped cilantro; or, 1-2 sprigs of curry leaves
one-thumb sized piece of fresh ginger, grated
1 tbsp cumin
1 tbsp black mustard seed
½ tsp hing powder
2 tbsp coriander powder
½-1 tsp turmeric
½-1 tsp black pepper
1-2 tsp pink salt (sanchal)
2-3 tbsp ghee

Directions
Melt ghee in a wok or large saucepan at medium heat, and when it begins to glisten add in fresh ginger, cumin and black mustard seed. If you are using curry leaf instead of cilantro, slide the leaves off the curry sprig and into the pan. When the mustard seeds just begin to pop, add in hing, coriander, turmeric, black pepper and pink salt. Stir for a half minute and then add in amaranth greens, turning the heat up a little higher. Cook veggies for about 2-3 minutes on high heat, then reduce it back to a medium heat. Continue to cook, stirring frequently, just until the leaves turn a bright, brilliant green. Serves 2-4 people.

For variations, use different herbs and spices. Have a little gas? Add some ajwain, crushed fenugreek seed or fennel seed. Maybe today the kapha is a little thick and heavy? Add in some red chili powder. Or instead of cilantro or curry leaf, try some Thai Basil instead.

Garlic-Basil Rapini

Rapini is a kind of turnip green, and like many of the healthful leafy greens, is found in the cruciferous family of vegetables. It is the Mediterranean version of the Chinese gai lan, and has a taste reminiscent of broccoli. For the best flavor, try to pick the rapini before the flowers have completely formed. This recipe capitalizes on the aromatic flavor of basil, which along with garlic, assists in digestion and boosts the immune system.

Ingredients
1 bunch of chopped rapini
5-6 cloves of minced garlic
1 small bunch of chopped fresh Italian basil
2 tbsp extra virgin olive oil
½ tsp salt

Directions
Over medium-low heat, add the olive oil and when it warms up, add in the chopped rapini and minced garlic. Stir-fry at medium heat and add the salt. Just as the rapini looks like it is done add in the chopped basil and stir-fry for another minute or two, until everything is bright green in color. Serves 2-4 people.

Ginger-Tamari Winter Squash

The Cucurbitaceae or gourd family has given us an amazingly diverse array of fruits to choose from, from the super-sweet watermelon to the intensely potent bitter gourd. In the northern hemisphere, autumn typically brings a huge abundance of winter squashes, including pumpkin, spaghetti, acorn, delicata, hubbard, buttercup and butternut squash. All have different flavors, some like pumpkin and hubbard are quite starchy, whereas others such as butternut and delicata are quite sweet by comparison. The following recipe can use any winter squash, but will obviously taste better with a sweeter-tasting squash.

Ingredients
1 large butternut squash
1 thumb-sized piece of grated fresh ginger

3-4 tbsp tamari
2 tbsp tahini

<u>Directions</u>
Split squash and remove seeds. Slice into one inch thick slabs or slices and placed on a lightly greased cookie sheet. In a separate bowl mix together grated ginger, tamari and tahini, and then using a soupspoon ladle sauce overtop squash. Bake at 350°F/175°C for approximately 45 minutes until the squash is lightly browned and fork tender. For an Indian variation on this recipe, prepare a sauce made with cinnamon, nutmeg, ginger, cardamom, black pepper and clove, mixed with a little jaggery and ghee. Serves 2-4 people, depending on the size of the squash.

Muttar Panir

Muttar panir is the classic Indian vegetarian dish of north India, made with fresh green peas and an Indian cheese called panir (p. 178), and is often eaten with flatbread (p. 186). It can be made in a variety of ways, with water or stock as the base, or by using cream or fermented cream products like crème fraîche to make a thick, luxurious sauce. Nowadays muttar panir is often made with tomatoes but they can be excluded from the recipe for people with sensitivities to the nightshade family.

The feature ingredient in this dish is pea (muttar), another member of the legume family. Fresh peas are quite different from dried peas, with a higher sugar content, fewer antinutrient factors, and much less in the way of protein. Peas contain a natural compound called m-xylohydroquinone that was studied in the 1950's for its contraceptive properties,[260] and perhaps due to its anti-estrogenic effects some practitioners find that peas help to reduce premenstrual syndrome. [261]

<u>Ingredients</u>
1 lb panir, chopped into chunks
1 onion, finely chopped
2 large tomatoes, cut into chunks
1 cup shelled green peas
1-2 tsp cumin seed
1 tsp ginger paste

1 tsp garlic paste
2 tsp coriander powder
½ tsp turmeric
5-6 crushed cardamom pods
1 inch cinnamon stick
2-3 cloves
½ tsp turmeric powder
½ - 1 tsp cayenne powder
¼ cup heavy cream
¼ cup water
2-3 tbsp ghee
¼ cup methi, finely chopped
¼ cup coriander, finely chopped
salt to taste

Directions
Melt one tbsp ghee and at medium heat fry the panir until golden and remove from heat. In a clean pan, add ghee and sauté the cumin seed and diced onion at medium-low heat until the onions are caramelized. Add in the garlic and ginger and the remaining herbs, spices and salt and sauté for five minutes. Add in the cream, mix well, and then add in enough water to make a thin sauce. Add the chopped tomatoes and cook uncovered until the sauce thickens. When it's ready, add in the green peas and panir, and cook for 5-10 minutes until the peas are bright green. Add the chopped methi and coriander and serve with freshly made flatbread (p. 186) or pullao (p. 183).

Fermented Vegetables

Old-fashioned Sauerkraut

Sauerkraut is the classic food of Eastern Europe, derived from the German term for 'soured cabbage'. Like many leafy greens the cabbage is a hybrid of the wild mustard *(Brassica oleracea)*, and its healing and medicinal virtues have long been extolled by the ancients. Of cabbage Cato the Elder claimed many uses: in the treatment of digestive disorders and colic, as well as arthritis, ulcers, nasal polyps, deafness and tumors, and applied topically as a poultice for wounds, sores and infection. In the 1950s, raw cabbage juice caught the attention of researchers, and was found to have anti-ulcer and anti-inflammatory effects in the digestive tract.[262] More recently, the sulfur containing compounds in cabbage including phenethyl isothiocyanate and sulforaphanehave been shown to have potent antioxidant and anti-tumor properties.[263]

Given the rather ubiquitous presence of cabbage and cabbage-like sisters including sui choy all over the world, it is no surprise there is such a diversity of live culture cabbage dishes, from the traditional European sauerkraut, to Kimchi (p. 161) in Korea. The following recipe favors the European palette, and contains herbs that are good for relieving gas and bloating, but can just as easily be left out for a simpler flavor.

Instructions
2 lbs grated cabbage (one cabbage head)
1 onion, chopped fine
1 tbsp salt
½ tsp dill seed
½ tsp savory seed
½ tsp coriander seed
½ tsp black pepper
½ tsp caraway seed

Directions
Mix grated cabbage and onion in a large, clean mixing bowl with clean hands, and add in the salt and herbs. Mix and gently

knead cabbage for about 5 minutes, ensuring that everything is well mixed. Stuff the cabbage into a clean, dry, large wide-mouth mason jar, pressing down on the mixture as you add each handful. Seal the jar and set it aside for 1-2 hours, and then with clean hands, push down on the mixture so that the liquid brine rises to the surface. Put aside for 2 days, and then open the jar to release the (stinky) gasses that accumulate. Reseal and set aside for 2 weeks and then enjoy, storing in the fridge to preserve the flavor and prevent it from becoming too sour.

Pickled Pepper Paste

Pickled peppers are a delightful way to preserve the huge diversity of bell peppers that are available in late summer, coming in a variety of colors, shapes and size. With high recommendations by Peter Piper, pickled peppers are a great way to eat probiotic foods, although with pickling it is very difficult to preserve the crispy crunch of a fresh bell pepper. Instead I use pickled peppers to make pepper paste, a tasty condiment that you can add to other dishes.

Ingredients
1 lb bell peppers, sliced
1 quart water
2 tbsp salt

Directions
Clean peppers and remove stem and core. Slice peppers in half and stuff into a clean jar. Dissolve the salt in the water and pour over top of the peppers. For variety add herbs such as basil and rosemary for a Mediterranean flavor, or chilies and garlic to get a spicy kick. Ensure that the peppers stay below the surface of the brine during fermentation, either by filling the jar all the way to the top, or by using a sterilized flat rock placed on top of the peppers to push everything down. On the second day open the jar to release all the carbon dioxide and reseal. Put aside for 2-3 weeks and then strain out the brine. Chop the peppers and then put them in the blender to make a paste. Store the paste in a clean dry jar in the fridge, and use within the next several weeks. With a little sugar or honey, pepper paste is a unique twist on catsup.

Kimchi

Just as there are a huge number of sauerkraut recipes, so too is there an enormous diversity of kimchi, the traditional pickle of Korea. Some recipes are as simple as cabbage and salt, whereas others are more complex, calling for non-vegetable ingredients such as fish. The following recipe is a delicious variation on traditional kimchi, using the pickled pepper paste (p. 160) to kick in fermentation. If you're not using the pepper paste, add in an extra tablespoon of salt.

Ingredients
1 head of sui choy cabbage, chopped
½ onion, chopped
1 thumb-sized piece of fresh ginger, grated
3-5 green onions, chopped
½ head of garlic, minced
2 cup of pickled pepper paste
½ - 1 tsp of crushed red chilies
1 tsp tamari
½ tsp fish sauce
1 tsp toasted sesame oil

Directions
Chop the vegetables and with clean hands mix them with all the other ingredients in a large mixing bowl. Do this for several minutes, ensuring that the red pepper paste is equally distributed. Stuff inside a clean dry jar and set aside for 1-2 weeks before refrigerating. This kimchi is excellent for kapha conditions and coldness, and to promote appetite and good circulation.

Carrot Pickle

Pickles are an important part of every culture and no less so in India. Unfortunately, most of the pickles that one can buy including Indian pickles are not the real deal, and are made with vinegar and sugar, rather than the fermented probiotic food they should be. Here is my variation on a traditional Indian carrot pickle.

Ingredients
2 lbs carrots
5-10 slices of fresh ginger
1 tsp cumin
1 tsp coriander
1 tsp black mustard
½ - 1 tsp dried crushed chili
2 tbsp salt
1 quart water

Directions

Wash carrots well and remove ends and tips. Slice in half length-wise, and then chop up carrots into finger-length slices, and stuff into a clean, dry mason jar. In a separate pan, dry roast the herbs on medium heat until the black mustard seed pops, and then pour them over the carrots. Dissolve the salt in the water and then pour this over the carrots. If you run out of brine, you can make another batch, using the ratio of 2 tbsp salt per quart water. Ensure that the carrots stay below the surface of the brine, either by filling the jar all the way to the top, or by using a clean, dry, flat rock that you previously sterilized, placed on top of the carrots to push everything down. On the second day open the jar to release all the carbon dioxide and reseal. From this point forward the carrot pickle can be eaten, but then by about the third week move the pickles to the fridge to slow down fermentation and preserve flavor.

Spicy Daikon Relish

The word 'relish' simply means something that adds flavor or zest, but in essence has traditionally been something used to enhance digestion. The artificially green, saccharine-sweet cucumber relish we all know was originally much more than a favored condiment for hot-dogs, it was a fermented pickle prepared with spicy and aromatic herbs to help digest the fattiness of farm-fresh sausage.

This recipe makes use of daikon, a root related to radish and rutabaga in the cruciferous family. Packed with antioxidant nutrients, daikon was traditionally used to enhance digestion, dispel mucus and enhance metabolism. Included as well are garlic, ginger and chili, making this a potent combination to power up the heat and reduce excess mucus (kapha).

The recipe is made in two stages: first, to make the daikon pickle, and then to make the relish. **Stage one** is as follows:

Ingredients
2 medium daikon roots, chopped
½ head of garlic, peeled and chopped
1 thumb-sized piece of ginger, chopped
1 tsp crushed dried chili
1 quart or liter of water
2 tbsp salt

Directions
Chop the daikon into finger-sized pieces and arrange in a jar, layering in the chili, ginger and garlic. When the jar is full, mix up a brine with the water and salt, pour over the daikon, cover and set aside for 2 weeks, making sure to release the gases that build up in the first couple days.

Stage two is making the relish. Hopefully you haven't eaten all the daikon pickle you made a few weeks ago, because it is pretty tempting on its own. Take what you have left and pour off the brine.

Ingredients
2 cups pickled daikon, chopped
½ red onion, finely chopped
4 medium tomatoes, chopped
2 large cucumbers, sliced into small pieces
1 bunch cilantro, chopped

Directions
Toss the ingredients together for a few minutes in a mixing bowl and then transfer to a jar. Eat immediately, or better yet, set aside on the counter for several days to let the vegetables ferment and flavors mix. Transfer to the refrigerator and enjoy over the next couple weeks. This relish is the perfect accompaniment to meat, egg and legume dishes.

Salsa

Salsa is the traditional condiment of Mexico, and is prepared in many different ways with a variety of ingredients. The key component of salsa is the tomatoes, including both red (roja salsa) tomatoes and green (verde salsa) tomatillos. In Mexico salsa is often made with fresh, cooked or canned ingredients. Salsa however can also be made into a delicious live culture food, providing the zesty flavor of Mexico and all the benefits of probiotic food.

Ingredients
2 lbs ripe tomato or tomatillos, finely chopped
1 red onion, finely chopped
2-4 fresh green chilies, diced
½ head garlic, diced
1 bunch of cilantro, finely chopped
2 tsp salt

Directions
Place all the ingredients in a large mixing bowl and add the salt. Mix well to distribute the salt. Pour contents into a clean dry jar and seal. Set aside for 2-3 days and periodically release the gas that accumulates. This salsa is ready to eat within 3-4 days, and after 1-2 weeks of fermentation can be stored in the refrigerator to preserve the flavor. Mix half and half with fresh avocado to make a delicious guacamole.

Add some variety by experimenting with different types of chili, such as chipotle, or add cooked black turtle beans to the mix. Consider adding in other vegetables or fruits such as chopped cabbage, carrot or mango, and experiment with different herbs such as oregano, rosemary, mint, black pepper and epazote.

Meat, Poultry and Fish

Five-Spice Bison Stew

Five-Spice is a key ingredient of Chinese food, and is usually a combination of aromatic, digestion-enhancing herbs such as star anise or fennel, Szechuan pepper, ginger, cinnamon and clove. These aromatic flavors help to counter the heavy qualities of the bison and promote good digestion. This recipe with its sweet flavor and medicinal herbs is particularly useful for reducing vata, in deficiency conditions such as infertility and weakness, as well as to promote good health during the cold and dry seasons. As a base formula, Five-Spice has many variations, often substituting in chili or black pepper for the harder to find Szechuan pepper or hua jiao *(Zanthoxylum bungeanum)*. Used in herbal medicine to promote circulation and to treat tooth problems, Szechuan pepper has a unique, tingly flavor that isn't quite as spicy as regular chili.

Ingredients
3-4 lbs bison stew meat
2 onions, cut into eighths
1 medium daikon root, chopped into 1 inch chunks
6-8 dried Chinese brown (shiitake) mushrooms
small handful of star anise seed pods
2-3 sticks of cinnamon
8-10 cloves
1 thumb-sized piece of fresh ginger root, thinly sliced
1 tsp fresh crushed black pepper and/or hua jiao
3 tbsp extra virgin sesame oil or pork fat
3-5 cloves of sliced garlic
½ tsp of toasted sesame oil
2 tbsp of tamari sauce
¼ cup molasses
2 cups of soup stock
1 small handful of Chinese red dates
5-6 slices of astragalus root
1 small handful of American ginseng root

<u>Directions</u>

In a medium sized bowl soak Chinese brown (shiitake) mushrooms in enough hot water to cover for about 10-15 minutes. In a skillet sauté star anise seed pods with cinnamon sticks, clove, ginger root and black pepper in sesame oil or pork fat, over a medium heat. Add in sliced garlic cloves and stewing meat, and mix well until the meat is lightly browned. Add in chopped onion and daikon root. Drain the soaking mushrooms, cut off the stems, slice into about ¼ inch segments and add to the stew. Stir this mixture constantly until the onions get a little translucent, and then add in tamari (soy) sauce, molasses, toasted sesame oil and soup stock. Add in Chinese red dates, astragalus root and American ginseng root, bring the stew to a boil then reduce to a simmer. If using a pressure cooker, cook for 45-60 minutes at 15 psi, and if using a regular pot, cook at low heat for approximately 2-3 hours, or until the meat is tender. Just before serving garnish with fresh chopped cilantro. Easily serves 4-5 people.

This recipe is adaptable to many different types of meats including lamb shanks, goat, mutton, beef or chicken.

Herb Poached Wild Salmon

Salmon has long been an important staple food eaten by coastal peoples along both the Pacific and Atlantic oceans. Since the collapse of the Atlantic salmon fishery decades ago, wild Atlantic salmon is hard to find, even though farmed Atlantic salmon from the Pacific Coast has become more common. Increasingly there have been concerns raised about the sustainability of farmed Atlantic salmon, everything from spreading disease to the wild salmon populations[264] as well as contamination from antibiotics,[265] heavy metals,[266] and PCBs.[267] While I typically counsel my patients to avoid farmed salmon I do recommend wild Pacific salmon. Due to the pollution of salmon spawning grounds as well as contaminants found in the ocean however, even the consumption of wild salmon should be limited to no more than twice a week.

Salmon is particularly rich in omega 3 fatty acids that are essential to the body and help regulate inflammation. In a recent study of traditional peoples living in northern Canada, a diet rich in salmon and fish fat was shown to reverse the progression of diabetes and cardiovascular disease.[268]   The highest fat content is found in the belly and just under the skin of the salmon, and overall, is highest in the king (Chinook) and sockeye salmon. Of the different species of salmon chum (dog) salmon has the lowest amount of fat, but because the fish spawns in intertidal waters and forages lower on the food chain, it likely contains the lowest levels of contaminants in its flesh.

I once heard a chef say that "you can never overcook salmon" – clearly this wasn't from someone who knew what they were talking about! To get the best flavor, salmon should be cooked using moist heat, and only to the point at which it begins to gently flake. It is possible to achieve this with baking or grilling, but it often requires added oils and sauces to preserve moisture. In my estimation there is nothing more disappointing than dry flakey salmon.

Ingredients
4 wild salmon steaks
1 tbsp fresh chopped dill herb
1 tbsp fresh chopped fennel herb
1 tbsp fresh chopped parsley
1 tbsp fresh chopped chives
1 tsp paprika
1 tsp salt
1 tsp black pepper
2-3 tbsp cultured butter
½ cup water, stock or white wine

Directions
In a large saucepan melt butter and sauté salmon steaks at a medium temperature until they become golden brown. Flip steaks and sprinkle herbs, pepper and salt over the fish. Add water or wine, reduce heat to a simmer and cover. Let cook for an additional 5-10 minutes until the salmon meat separates into large wedges of gelatinous salmony goodness. Serves four people.

Mexican Chicken Stew

Mexican cuisine is a unique blend of flavors that mixes Old World herbs such as garlic, oregano, cumin, cinnamon and lime, with distinctly Central American representatives such as smoked chili (chipotle), epazote, and annatto seed (achiote). With its reliance upon soupy stews and legume dishes, Mexican cuisine is in many ways similar to Indian cuisine, relying on a highly flavored mixture of spices and herbs called a mole that resembles the masala spice mixtures used in India.

This recipe calls for the chipotle pepper, which derives its unique flavor from carefully smoking the chili over different types of wood including mesquite, hickory, oak and other hardwoods. Although ripe jalapeño peppers are typically used, a variety of other peppers can be dried and smoked for this purpose including the relatively mild pasilla pepper, the hotter morita and serrano peppers, and the catecholamine-pumping habañero. Smoking the chili peppers reduces the intensity of heat by about 20-30%, and adds an earthy, smoky flavor that is distinct to Mexican cuisine. If you can't get chipotle, you can try making your own chili powder by dry roasting cayenne pepper with other herbs such as paprika, cinnamon, nutmeg, clove and black pepper. Chili peppers are excellent to enhance digestion, eliminate congestion (kapha) and promote good circulation, but are contraindicated in excess heat (pitta) or dryness (vata).

This recipe also calls for epazote, a relative of lambsquarters and a frequent weed of Mexican gardens. It has an aromatic flavor reminiscent of gasoline or paint thinner, but when cooked yields more of a citrusy herb flavor. It is used to enhance the digestion of legumes, and is excellent to prevent and rid the body of parasites, which are more common in warmer climates like Mexico.

Ingredients
1 whole chicken
2 onions, chopped
2-3 stalks celery, chopped
6 roma tomatoes, chopped
1 head garlic, minced
2 tbsp dried oregano
2 tbsp paprika
1 tbsp dried basil
1-2 tsp dried epazote
1 tsp cumin seed
2-3 dried bay leaves

2-5 chipotle dried peppers, finely chopped
1 tsp salt
1 tsp black pepper
2-3 tbsp olive oil
cilantro, as garnish
goat feta, as garnish

Directions

In a pressure cooker at medium heat, sauté onions and celery, and add in garlic, oregano, paprika, basil, epazote, cumin seed, chipotle peppers, salt and pepper. Cook until onions are translucent and add in tomatoes. Move all the vegetables to the side of the pot and place the whole chicken in the center. Add in 2-3 cups of chicken stock and the bay leaves. Cover pressure cooker, bring to a boil and then cook under highest pressure for 60-80 minutes. This can also be cooked in a Dutch oven for approximately 2-3 hours at 350°F/180°C. Before serving, use a spoon to break the chicken into small pieces and remove the large bones. Serve with freshly made tortillas and/or rice, and garnish with crumbled goat feta and chopped cilantro.

Goat Curry

According to Ayurveda, goat meat is one of the few types of meat that is suitable to all three doshas, a virtue seemingly understood by peoples throughout Asia, making it one of the most commonly consumed meats. For one thing, goat meat brings none of the religious baggage of other meats, and is equally consumed by almost all peoples, including Hindus, Muslims, Jews and Christians. From a nutritional perspective, goat meat is very dense in nutrients, especially when prepared as a stew, which usually includes bone and marrow. Being curious browsers rather than focused grazers, goats consume a broader array of plant foods and nutrients than ruminants like beef or bison, which may explain why goat meat has a more balancing, harmonizing effect. Pasture-raised goat meat can often be found at halal and East Indian butchers.

The following recipe is a basic curry, for which any meat can be used, adjusting the cooking time as needed. Likewise, the mixture of herbs called the masala can vary depending on the flavors desired. This recipe has a mixture of sweet, bitter and pungent flavors, which has a balancing, harmonious effect in the body.

Ingredients
3-4 lbs goat meat, bone in
2 onions, finely chopped
2-3 stalks celery, finely chopped
2 medium zucchinis, in large 1 inch chunks
2 tsp cumin seed
1 tsp black mustard seed
2-3 tsp coriander seed powder
½ tsp turmeric
½ tsp fenugreek seed
10 cardamom pods, crushed
2-3 sticks of cinnamon
6-8 cloves
6-8 garlic cloves, chopped
1 thumb-sized piece of fresh ginger, grated
1 sprig of curry leaves, separated from stem
1 tsp black pepper
1 tsp pink salt (sanchal)
2-3 tbsp ghee
2 cups soup stock

Directions
In a large heavy-bottom pot, sauté the cumin, black mustard, fenugreek, cardamom, cinnamon and cloves in ghee over a medium heat. As the mustard seed begins to pop, add in the coriander seed powder, turmeric and pink salt. Add in garlic, ginger, and goat meat. Brown the meat in the spices and ghee for about 5-10 minutes and then add onions, celery and zucchini, and cook until the onions become a little translucent. Add in enough soup stock to cover, bring to a boil, reduce to a simmer and cook at low heat for 3-4 hours, or 1 hour in a pressure cooker at 15 psi. Approximately 10-15 minutes before serving, sauté fresh curry leaves with fresh crushed black pepper in a tablespoon of ghee at medium heat, for several minutes, but do not blacken. When the goat stew is done, remove the lid and add in the curry leaf and black pepper mixture, and allow to infuse into the stew for several minutes before serving. Serves four or more people.

Persian Lamb Shanks

Persian lamb shanks are the quintessential comfort food of Iran and Persian cuisine, a popular time-honored dish that is cooked in every home. Given where Iran is located in western Asia, it might be expected that Persian cuisine is a hybrid of both Indian and European flavors, using Indian herbs such as black cumin and ginger along with more conventionally European herbs such as parsley and dill. The combination is a fragrant admixture of delicate aromas that is uniquely Persian and totally delicious. To boost the medicinal quality add in a few slices of dang gui and peony root, two important Chinese herbs to nourish the blood to treat infertility. The dang gui in particular has a strong celery flavor that complements this dish nicely.

Lamb shanks are the forelimbs of the lamb, rich in sinewy tendons and muscle, and like many tough or stringy meats, needs to be braised with moist heat (see p. 118). In medicinal terms, lamb shanks are good for building up the sinewy muscles and bones, and are a particularly good food for balancing vata.

Ingredients
4 lamb shanks
2 - 4 cups of stock
4 stalks of finely chopped celery
1 finely chopped onion
½ head of finely chopped garlic
2-3 tbsp butter, olive oil or ghee
1 tsp black cumin
1 tbsp of dried leek leaf
1 tbsp of dried parsley leaf
1 tbsp of dried dill leaf
1 tbsp of dried mint leaf
1 tsp of sea salt
fresh-cracked black pepper, as garnish
fresh cilantro, as garnish

Directions
On medium-low heat, lightly brown the lamb shanks in butter or ghee, and then set aside. Add a little more fat to the pot and add in onion, garlic, celery, cumin, leek, parsley, dill and mint. Stir-fry until onions are translucent, and then add the lamb

shanks, stock and salt. If you are using a pressure cooker, use only two cups of stock, whereas if you are making it in a heavy cast iron pot use four cups of water, and cook covered at low heat for 3-4 hours. Garnish with fresh cracked black pepper and cilantro. Serves four or more people.

Dhaniya Chicken

When you are pressed for time and don't have the ability to do more, Dhaniya Chicken holds itself out as a simple way to prepare a delightful dish with a minimum amount of fuss. The primary flavor here is dhaniya, or coriander seed, which has a distinctive lemon flavor that instantly jazzes up any savory dish. Coriander seed is one the best medicines in Ayurveda to relieve gas, bloating and digestive upset, helping to stimulate the liver and reduce pitta and inflammation. Dhaniya alleviates all three doshas, enhances digestion and benefits the heart. It is particularly rich in minerals such as calcium, iron, magnesium and manganese.

Ingredients
1 chicken, whole or chopped
1 onion, chopped
2-3 tbsp coriander seed (dhaniya) powder
1 tsp salt
1 tsp black pepper
½ tsp turmeric

Directions
Place the chicken and onion in a baking dish and add the herbs, sprinkling over a whole chicken, or mixing into the chopped chicken. Bake at 350°F/175°C for 60-80 minutes. For more of a punch, add in a ½ tsp hing and 1 tsp of dried red chili pepper. This recipe can also be adapted to other dishes such as lamb kabobs, grilled meat and vegetarian dishes such as baked tofu or roasted vegetables. Garnish with fresh-chopped cilantro.

Dairy

Boiled Milk

Boiled milk is a favored food and home remedy all over the world, and is an excellent medium to extract the medicinal properties of different herbs. On its own boiled milk is heavier and harder to digest than fresh raw milk, but by using certain digestive-enhancing herbs we can offset this effect. These include the common chai masala spices including ginger, cardamom, cinnamon, clove, fennel and black pepper.

The basic method to boil milk is to scald it, cooking the milk on medium-low, bringing the temperature of the milk up to about 185°F/85°C. Stir the milk frequently so that the surface doesn't form a thick skin and it doesn't burn. When the milk begins to boil, reduce to a simmer, and allow the milk to cook for another 5 minutes. Prepared in this fashion boiled milk has a heavy and warm quality, and helps to relax the body and quiet the mind. Ghee can be mixed into boiled milk to enhance its nourishing properties, used in weakness, infertility, exhaustion and during post-partum. Finely powdered herbs can also be added in and cooked for 5-10 minutes on low heat, filtering the resultant liquid with a metal mesh strainer. To make a more efficient extract however dilute the milk with an equal part water, bring it to a boil and then simmer on low until all or most of the water is gone. This prevents the milk from burning, allows for a longer decoction to make a stronger extract, and makes the final preparation easier to digest. Any number of herbs can be added to boiled milk to change or modify its properties. The doses for the following herbs are based on a one cup (250 mL) serving:

- Turmeric: dry cough, bronchitis, arthritis and skin problems; ½ -1 tsp of the powdered rhizome
- Ginger: nausea, indigestion, spasm, headache; ½ -1 tsp of the powdered rhizome
- Nutmeg: muscle pain, insomnia, poor libido; ¼ tsp of the fresh ground fruit
- Cardamom: excess mucus, indigestion, headache; 4-8 crushed pods

- Fennel: nausea, indigestion, insufficient lactation; 1 tsp of the crushed seed
- Ashwagandha: fatigue, stress, insomnia, infertility; 1 tbsp of the powdered root
- Shatavari: burning sensations, ulcers, infertility; 1 tbsp of the powdered root
- Bala: stress, weakness, exhaustion, infertility; 1 tbsp of the powdered root
- Garlic: arthritis, back pain and cardiovascular disease; 1 tsp of the fresh minced bulb
- Licorice: colds, bronchitis, asthma; 1 tsp of the powdered root
- Arjun: bronchitis, diarrhea, cardiovascular disease; 1 tsp of the powdered bark
- Dates, figs, raisins, goji: anemia, fatigue, infertility, weakness; 1-2 tbsp chopped fruit

With the exception of dried fruit milk decoctions, sweeteners are sometimes added to milk decoctions to modify a medicinal effect. The most common sweetener used in Ayurveda is jaggery (gur), added in during the last stages of cooking to give the milk a cooling quality. Other sweeteners such as malts and syrups can be added in the same fashion, but honey should only be added once the milk has cooled to room temperature.

Homemade Yogurt

Yogurt, or dahi as it is called in India and Nepal, is a food consumed and relished by milk-drinking cultures all over the world. Simply meaning 'sour milk' in Turkish, what we call yogurt has come to refer to a type of fermented milk preparation that has been inoculated with specific bacterial strains including *Lactobacillus bulgaricus* and *Streptococcus thermophilus*. Held at room temperature, raw milk will eventually culture due to the presence of naturally occurring bacteria and yeasts, but the final product can vary considerably in consistency and flavor. To properly control fermentation, yogurt is best made with the assistance of live culture yogurt, or a starter made from freeze-dried, frozen or spray-dried bacteria.

Ingredients
1 liter milk
4 tbsp fresh live culture plain yogurt, or
yogurt starter (follow manufacturers directions)

Directions

Filter the raw milk through some cheesecloth or a metal mesh strainer to remove any particulate or impurities. Place in a pot and scald the milk, let it simmer for five minutes, and then pour the hot milk into a clean dry mason jar to cool. Cool the milk until it's just warm, and add in the live culture yogurt or yogurt starter. Seal with a lid and give it a shake to mix. Put the jar aside in a warm location for 8-10 hours, and then refrigerate immediately to preserve the sweetness of the yogurt.

The optimal temperature for culturing yogurt is about 110°F/43°C, which should be maintained for at least 2-3 hours before gradually cooling to room temperature. There are a variety of methods used to maintain this temperature, and much of the concern relates to the ambient temperature. In hot climates or during the summer nothing more is required than wrapping the jar in a towel and letting it sit on the counter. In cool weather, turn the oven on to its lowest setting, and place the towel-wrapped jar on the stove for a couple hours before turning it off. If you want to use smaller jars for single servings, pour the inoculated milk into several small mason jars and then place these in a cooler along with a jar of boiling hot water, which keeps the interior of the cooler nice and warm.

One of the most frequent uses for yogurt in India is to make *raita*, or yogurt salad. Vegetables such as cucumber and cilantro are mixed with roasted spices such as cumin, coriander, turmeric, black pepper and salt. In much the same fashion, Greek *tatziki* is made with cucumber, a little minced garlic, and herbs such as black pepper, parsley and salt. In Iran the local variation there is called *masto khiar*, and is made with ingredients such as chopped cucumber, crushed walnuts and soaked raisins, and garnished with fresh herbs such as mint leaf. When the weather gets really hot, my favorite drink is to dilute yogurt with cool water and blend with fresh mint, rose petals and a little sugar. Many different things can be made with yogurt, but according to Ayurveda there are some foods that are incompatible with yogurt such as sour-tasting fruit, meat and legumes (p. 29). For more information on the general properties of yogurt, please review the earlier section on dairy (p. 61).

Cultured Butter

Most of the butter people eat nowadays is creamery butter, which is butter made from fresh cream. It has a predictably bland, sweet taste very unlike the rich pungent flavor of cultured butter. While creamery butter has its uses, for most of our history humans have almost always eaten cultured butter instead. The primary reason for this is that soured cream is far easier to churn into butter than fresh cream. The side benefit apart from the distinct flavor is that cultured butter is a probiotic food, making it easier to digest than conventional butter. According to Ayurveda cultured butter is a natural rejuvenative (rasayana), and helps to balance both vata and pitta. In contrast, creamery butter is more difficult to digest, and facilitates the production of kapha and ama.

On a traditional dairy farm the process of making cultured butter begins by skimming the cream off the fresh raw milk, and then setting it aside at room temperature (68°F/20°C) to culture. Letting the cream sit for a day or so produces a relatively mild-tasting butter, whereas letting it sit for several days produces a much stronger flavor.

If you can't get access to raw milk or cream, cultured butter can also be made from pasteurized cream. Look for the highest percent fat content you can find (33% or more), making sure that the only ingredient is 100% cream (i.e. with no milk solids, stabilizers or flavors added). Scald the cream using the same method as boiled milk (p. 173) and let it cool to room temperature. To ferment the cream, use either a sour cream starter or use 1 tbsp of commercial sour cream or buttermilk per cup of cream. Mix into a clean dry jar and let sit for 2-3 days, tasting it periodically with a clean, dry spoon to get the desired flavor.

Once the cream has fermented, the water and proteins must be separated out to make the butter. To do this the soured cream needs to be churned, forcefully breaking apart the molecular structure of the cream to allow the butterfat to congeal, leaving behind the buttermilk. Many methods can be used to churn butter, from the simple wooden churners still used in developing countries, to the large electric churners used in commercial dairy operations. At home either an empty mason jar or a regular kitchen blender is all the equipment that's needed.

Before churning the butter, reduce the temperature of the cream to between 50-60°F (10-15°C), which optimizes the ability of the butterfat to congeal. You can do this by putting the jar of soured cream in a bowl of cold water, or if it's cool outside set it on the porch. If using the "jar method", add the sour cream to the jar until it's half-full and shake vigorously for 15-20 minutes or more. If using a blender, mix the sour cream for about 5-10 minutes on medium speed, after which time the butter and buttermilk will have separated. Pour off the buttermilk and set it aside for later use. Put the butter in a bowl and add cold water to the butter, mixing and working the butter with a wooden spoon to remove any remaining buttermilk. Pour off the water, add some more cold water and repeat until the water is clear. Drain well, and the butter is now ready to use or can be rendered into ghee (p. 194). To preserve the butter for storage, add in between 1-3% sea salt, which for one pound (454 g) of butter is approximately 1 tsp (6 g). Make sure to mix in the salt well so that it is evenly distributed.

Khadi

Among the various foods that can be prepared from dairy, buttermilk is a unique medicinal food that is highly prized in Ayurveda. Unlike the thick gooey buttermilk in grocery stores, real buttermilk is a thin acidic liquid that separates out when churning butter. Called 'takra' in Sanskrit, real buttermilk is exceptionally useful to restore digestion and is used in Ayurveda as a treatment for many different conditions including fever, diarrhea and hemorrhoids. It is most frequently given as a medicinal soup called khadi, consumed on its own as a warm beverage, or mixed and eaten with rice. Khadi is an excellent food for any kind of indigestion, and is a very good food to restore digestion after fasting, or when recuperating from fever and diarrhea.

<u>Ingredients</u>
2-3 cups buttermilk

1 tsp cumin seed
1 tsp black mustard seed
½ tsp hing
½ tsp fenugreek seed
½ tsp turmeric powder
½ tsp black pepper
½ tsp salt
1 sprig of curry leaves, separated from stem
1 tbsp ghee

<u>Directions</u>
Melt the ghee in a pot at medium heat and add the cumin, black mustard and fenugreek seeds. When the mustard begins to pop add in the hing, turmeric, curry leaves and salt. Roast the herbs for another few minutes, and then add in the buttermilk. Bring to a boil, simmer for 5-10 minutes and then serve on its own as a soup, or mix with rice. For a variation, add in vegetables such as onion, garlic, zucchini, okra or tomato. To thicken the khadi add in 1-2 tablespoons of chickpea (besan) flour that has been premixed with a little cold water, and cook for another 10-15 minutes. In India khadi is most frequently eaten as an accompaniment to balance the intense flavor of hot, spicy dishes.

Panir

Panir is an unripened cheese that is made by separating out the casein-rich curds from the whey protein liquid. It requires the use of an acid medium such as lime or lemon to curdle the milk, and separate it into curds and whey.

<u>Ingredients</u>
2 quarts (one liter) milk
2-3 tbsp lime juice

<u>Directions</u>
Bring the milk to a boil, reduce the heat to low and add the limejuice, stirring continuously. Within a few minutes small curds rise to the surface. Continue stirring for about five minutes, waiting for the curds get larger and the surrounding whey to become more opaque. When done, turn off the heat and let

stand for few more minutes. Take a length of muslin cloth or cheesecloth and line a colander so that the cloth hangs over the edges of the colander. Place the colander in an empty sink and pour the curdled milk into it. Gather up the edges of the cheesecloth and tie the cloth onto the faucet, and allow the whey to drip out for about 30 minutes. Untie the cloth, gather up the edges and squeeze tightly, twisting the edges of the cloth to remove the remaining whey. Let it hang again for another hour or more to get a much firmer cheese. Store in the refrigerator and use within a couple days. It is good as a snack food, but has a rather bland taste, and is best used stir-fried with greens vegetables (e.g. saag panir) or in stews (see p. 157).

A variation on panir can be made with yogurt. Drain the yogurt with cheesecloth overnight by hanging it on the faucet of the sink, and when done squeeze well to remove any remaining liquid.

Grains and Legumes

Kitchari

Kitchari is the classical Ayurvedic panacea, eaten whenever there is ill health or during a therapeutic regimen such as panch karma and detoxification. Essentially made from rice, kitchari is a universal food found in other cultures, with similar sounding names such as 'kushari' in the Middle East and 'congee' in China. There are an infinite array of variations, and based on the herbs and spices chosen, can be prepared to reduce vata, pitta or kapha. The following recipe is definitely more Indian-inspired, using herbs and spices to enhance digestion. Prepared with whole grain mung and brown rice, kitchari has a more detoxifying effect.

Ingredients
1 cup brown basmati rice (fermented, p. 126)
1 cup green mung dhal (fermented, p. 126)
8-10 cups water
2 tbsp ghee
2 tsp cumin
2-3 cinnamon sticks, broken into large pieces
10-12 cardamom pods, crushed
1 tsp whole black pepper
½ tsp hing powder
½ tsp turmeric powder
sea salt, to taste

Directions
Ferment (p. 126) the rice and mung beans and drain before use. In a large pot melt ghee over medium heat and add in cumin, cinnamon bark, cardamom pods, black pepper, hing, turmeric and salt. Stir for a few minutes and then add in rice and dhal, cooking for a few more minutes before adding in 8 cups water or stock. Bring to a boil, reduce to a simmer and cook for 2-3 hours until the rice and dhal is soft. Whole grain kitchari is not necessarily ideal for those with weak digestion, and can be

substituted with white basmati rice and washed mung dhal. Soak 1-2 hours and drain for before use.

Asian kitchari is a variation on this recipe, substituting short grain brown rice for basmati rice, and adzuki bean for mung. Follow the same recipe but use flavors such as fresh ginger, garlic, seaweed and tamari. When it's done mix in a couple tablespoons of miso paste and garnish with fresh chopped shiso leaf or cilantro.

Urad Mung Dhal

Among the different beans recommended by Ayurveda, urad or black gram is considered to be unique, with heavy, warm and wet properties, making it the most nourishing of the legumes. Apart from the non-food legumes such as kapikacchu *(Mucuna pruriens)* and bu gu zhi *(Psoralea corylifolia)*, urad is the only bean used as a sexual restorative and aphrodisiac. The problem with urad however, is that it is difficult to digest and so needs to be properly prepared with herbs and spices or used with other beans such as mung to offset its heavy properties. This recipe calls for the use of washed whole beans, which have the skin coats washed off to promote digestion. Both the urad and the mung dhal should be dry roasted before use, stirring in a pan for 5-7 minutes on medium heat (p. 121).

Ingredients
½ cup urad dhal (roasted)
½ cup mung dhal (roasted)
1 thumb-sized piece of ginger, chopped into chunks
six cups water and/or soup stock
1 tsp cumin seed
1 tsp black mustard seed
½ tsp ajwain seed
1 tbsp coriander powder
2-3 bay leaves
½ tsp hing powder
½ tsp turmeric
1 tsp fresh ground black pepper
4-5 fresh chopped tomatoes
2 tsp salt
fresh cilantro

After roasting, soak the mung and urad in cool water for 20 minutes and then rinse. Add beans, water, ginger, bay leaves and salt to a medium pot, bring to a boil and reduce to a simmer, cooking for 1-2 hours. If using a pressure cooker, use less water and cook for 30-40 minutes at 15 psi. When the beans are almost cooked, in a separate pan, melt ghee and add cumin, black mustard and ajwain, and cook until the mustard seeds pop. Add in coriander powder, hing, turmeric and 1 tsp salt. Cook for another half minute or so, and then add in the chopped tomatoes, stir-frying at medium heat until the tomatoes are bright red and greasy looking. Add this mixture to the beans, and cook for another five minutes. Garnish with fresh chopped cilantro, and eat with freshly made rice and vegetables. Serves four people, eaten with rice or another grain dish.

This basic recipe can be adapted to any bean, including toor dhal, chana dhal, kidney beans, dried peas, moth and black-eyed peas. Instead of Indian flavoring consider the Mexican or Italian masalas described on page 142.

Breakfast Bowl

I typically recommend to most of my patients that they eat a high protein, high-fat breakfast, which is better suited to providing them with a stable energy source throughout the day. Most of the time these range from foods like eggs and vegetables, to fish or meat, but sometimes these foods are too heavy or warming. This recipe is a nice alternative to my typical recommendations, and is ideally suited to the summer months when the fire element tends to become over-balanced, requiring foods that are less heating in nature.

Ingredients
1 cup whole grain, e.g. brown rice, quinoa, buckwheat (fermented, p. 126)
2 cups water
¼ tsp salt
1 quarter chopped, medium cucumber
2 handfuls of sprouts, e.g. alfalfa, broccoli, onion
1 finely grated carrot
2 handfuls chopped leafy greens, e.g. arugula, romaine, radicchio

2 tbsp tahini
1 tsp tamari
hemp hearts (hulled hemp seeds), as a garnish

Directions
Add fermented grain, water and salt to a medium pot, bring to a boil and reduce to a simmer. Cook the grain for the required amount of time. Chop all the vegetable ingredients and place into a bowl. When it's done add the hot, freshly cooked grain over top of the raw vegetables. Mix up the tahini and tamari in a measuring cup, and pour over top of the grains, mixing well. The hot grains help cook the raw vegetables, making them more digestible. Garnish with hemp hearts to boost protein and fat content. Serves two.

Brown Basmati Pullao

Pullao is the classic rice dish of Indian cookery, prepared with soup stock and any number of herbs and spices. While white rice is more commonly consumed in India this is a relatively recent trend, and at one time all the rice consumed in India was either brown or partially milled rice. Referred to as mahasali in Ayurveda, basmati rice is unique among the different varietals of rice, not necessarily because it is considered to be the healthiest, but because it has a delightful nutty aroma and flavor. From a strict Ayurvedic perspective, the best rice to eat is raktasali, or red rice, of which there are a number of different varieties depending on location. Another medicinal rice is black rice, often called 'forbidden rice', because at one time its great virtues were reserved only for the local rulers. Both red and black rice are rich in antioxidant pigments such as cyanidin 3-glucoside.

Pullao is the perfect accompaniment to stewed meat dishes, beans and vegetables. The following recipe is a nutritious variation on an old theme:

Ingredients
2 cups brown basmati rice (fermented, p. 126)
1 tsp cumin seed
10-12 cardamom pods, crushed
6-8 cloves
2-3 cinnamon sticks, broken into chunks

¼ cup crushed almonds
¼ cup raisins
2 tbsp ghee
½ lemon, juiced
saffron, pinch
½ tsp salt
4 cups soup stock

Directions

Melt ghee in a pot and add the cumin, cardamom, cloves, cinnamon, crushed almonds and raisins. Stir-fry the ingredients in the ghee at a medium heat for a minute before adding in the rice. Continue frying the brown rice in the ghee for several minutes until the rice looks parched. Add in soup stock, lemon juice and salt. Bring to a boil and reduce to a simmer. Sprinkle the saffron on top and cook covered for 45 minutes. Toss well before serving. Serves 4-5 people.

There are a number of variations on this theme. I am also quite fond of Persian cuisine, and use herbs such as dried leek, dill weed and parsley, along with walnuts and mulberries. And instead of using rice, try other whole grains such as amaranth, barley or buckwheat (kasha).

Goji Quinoa Pilaf

Pilaf is Turkish for the Hindi word pullao, and thus using the word "pilaf" for this dish might be stretching it a bit, as a pilaf is typically made with rice. With the popularity of newer grains like quinoa, as well as the rediscovery of forgotten friends like buckwheat and barley, I take the term 'pilaf' to mean pretty much any grain dish prepared with stock, herbs, vegetables and spices. Originally grown by the Inca, quinoa in particular is an exceptional grain with a high protein content and no gluten, making it an ideal food for those with wheat allergies. This relatively straight-forward pilaf takes advantage of the healing properties of goji berries (gou zi), which in Chinese medicine are nourishing to the blood, liver and eyes.

Ingredients
2 cups quinoa (fermented, p. 126)
1 medium onion, diced

2 small handfuls of goji berries
2 tbsp oil (sesame, butter or olive)
4 cups stock
½ tsp salt

<u>Directions</u>
Melt butter in a pot at medium-low heat and sauté diced onions until caramelized. Add in the quinoa and cook for 5 minutes with the onions, then adding in the goji berries, cooking for another minute or so. Add the soup stock and salt, bring to a boil and simmer covered for 20 minutes. Toss before serving. Serves 4-5 people.

Northwest Wild Rice Infusion

Wild rice is a species of rice native to North America and China that is distantly related to what we conventionally called rice *(Oryza sativa)*. Now cultivated in Canada and elsewhere for the retail market, wild rice *(Zizania palustris)* is higher in protein and fiber than regular brown rice, and has a unique flavor and chewy texture. The following recipe calls for cranberries, which contain a number of beneficial antioxidants and anti-inflammatory compounds.

<u>Ingredients</u>
1 cup wild rice (fermented, p. 126)
1 cup long grain brown rice (fermented, p. 126)
¼ cup crushed hazelnuts
¼ cup dried cranberries (sugar-free)
½ tsp salt
2 tbsp butter
4 cups soup stock

<u>Directions</u>
Melt butter in a pot and add the rice, hazelnuts and cranberries. Stir-fry the ingredients for a couple minutes, and then add the soup stock and salt. Bring to a boil and reduce to a simmer. Cover and let cook for 45-50 minutes. Mix well before serving. Serves 4-5 people.

Indian Flatbread

There are many different types of Indian flatbread including roti (chapatti), thepla and parantha. The primary advantage of flatbread over conventional bread is that it's easier to digest, and doesn't have the same sticky and heavy properties as baked loaves. Roti is a plain Indian flatbread traditionally made with a stone-ground wheat flour called atta. Thepla is similar but thicker than roti, often made with different grains such as chana (chickpea) or millet, and usually includes herbs such as chopped fresh methi (fenugreek) or cilantro kneaded into the flour. A third type of Indian flatbread is parantha, which is usually stuffed with vegetables and herbs.

To make plain **roti**, follow these directions:

Ingredients
1 cup flour, germinated (p. 116) and roasted (p. 121)
1 cup sourdough culture (p. 127)
olive oil

Directions
Grind the flour to the desired consistency using a coffee grinder or a grain mill. Mix the flour and sourdough culture together, adding in a little water as required, and knead well. Place in a bowl and drizzle a little olive oil over the surface of the dough to keep it moist. Cover with a wet cloth and let sit for several hours in a warm place and let it ferment (2-18 hours). After fermentation, knead the dough again, and then break off pieces of the dough about the size of a golf ball, roll into a ball and put aside. Warm a large cast iron pan to medium heat with no oil. Sprinkle some flour onto a large flat surface such as a cutting board or a counter, and roll out each ball until it is a round, thin disc, and immediately place in the pan. Cook for approximately 1-2 minutes on each side. When golden brown, take the roti out of the pan and then place them on a hot burner very briefly until they puff up. Serves 3-4 people.

To make **thepla** use the same basic technique as roti, but add in the following ingredients after making the dough:

Ingredients
half cup fresh chopped methi (fenugreek)

2 tbsp sesame oil
1 tbsp sesame seeds
1 tsp ajwain seeds
1 tsp turmeric powder
½ tsp cracked black pepper
1 tsp salt

To make **parantha** prepare in the same manner as roti, but instead of mixing the ingredients into the flour, you are going to stuff the roti. For the filling many different vegetables can be used, including cabbage, broccoli and sweet potato, but my favorite is **gobi parantha** – made with cauliflower ('gobi').

Ingredients
1 small head of cauliflower, coarsely grated and drained
1 tsp cumin seed
1 tsp black mustard
½ tsp crushed coriander seed
½ tsp hing
½ tsp ajwain
½ tsp black pepper
½ tsp chili pepper
¼ tsp turmeric
½ tsp salt
2 tsp ghee

Directions
Grate the cauliflower (or any other vegetable), add the salt and mix well in a bowl. Let sit for 5 minutes then take a handful out at a time, squeezing out the excess liquid and put aside. Melt 1 tsp of ghee in a saucepan and roast the cumin, black mustard, coriander and ajwain for a minute until the mustard starts to pop, then add in the hing, turmeric and black pepper. Mix for a few seconds then add in the cauliflower. Stir-fry for a few minutes then put aside, half-cooked. Follow the recipe for roti: roll out each ball to about three inches in diameter, and place about 2 tbsp of filling in the middle. Make a dumpling by pulling the edges of the roti together, and then roll flat to no more than ¼ inch thickness. Parantha can also be made by rolling out two roti, laying the filling on one, covering with the second, pinching the edges closed and then rolling flat. Melt 1

tsp of ghee in a frying pan on medium-low heat, and fry each parantha on both sides until golden brown.

Rosemary Oatcakes

Ask any Scotsman and he will stand by the virtue of the mighty oat, some even insisting that they have a long and venerable past in Scotland – despite the fact that oats are originally native to the Mediterranean. Regardless of the real history, the oat is nonetheless an important staple for the people of Scotland, who learned to make use of seaweed as a natural manure that allowed them to grow oats and other grains in a place which otherwise has very little topsoil, increasing yields by 20-30 times. This recipe is made with the help of a sourdough, yielding flavored oatcakes that are more like a cracker than a pancake, meant to be eaten as a savory item along with foods such as sharp cheeses, cured meats and pickles.

Ingredients
1 cup sourdough starter
1 cup ground oatmeal
1 tbsp coarsely ground rosemary
1-2 tsp coarsely ground black pepper
1 tsp salt

Directions
Mix the starter and the ground oats, adding in the rosemary, black pepper and salt. Knead well, and then put aside for several hours to ferment. Knead again, and then roll out the dough to about one-eighth of an inch, cutting circular cakes about 2 ½ inches in diameter (a water glass works well). Lightly coat a baking sheet with butter and then lay the cakes out evenly on the pan. Bake at 300°F/150°C for 15 minutes or until golden brown.

For variation add in other herbs such as basil or oregano, or seaweed and sesame seed. They can also be made into sweet cakes by adding jaggery, as well as herbs and spices such as cinnamon and nutmeg. These oatcakes usually have a good shelf life, and are a high-energy food that is good for picnics, travel and camping.

Nuts and Seeds

Gomashio

Gomashio is a traditional Japanese condiment prepared from roasted sesame seed and sea salt that has been popularized by the macrobiotic food movement. It is the macrobiotic version of ketchup, a tasty and mouth-watering condiment that makes just about anything taste good. To make gomashio easily, use a special Japanese mortar and pestle called a suribachi. The mortar of the surabachi is a clay bowl with a roughened grinding surface carved into it, and the pestle is made of wood. This makes it very easy to grind soft herbs and seeds into a paste, which have a habit of jumping around when using a smooth-surfaced mortar and pestle.

Ingredients
8 tbsp whole sesame seed
1 tbsp sea salt

Directions
Roast the sesame seeds for 5-6 minutes at 250°F/120°C. Allow to cool and transfer to the surabachi. Add the sea salt and grind into a medium fine powder. Bottle and store in a cool, dry place. Make fresh each week.

For diversity, when roasting the sesame seeds add other herbs such as kelp, dulse, savory, nettle seed, cumin, coriander, black pepper or hing. Although gomashio is a Japanese dish it can easily married to other cuisines and flavors, serving not only a tasty condiment but a useful medicine to enhance digestion and boost mineral status. In Ayurveda, sesame seeds are used to boost energy, strengthen the hair and skin, counter deficiency and treat problems associated with vata.

Coconut Chutney

If I had to live on a deserted tropical island and could only bring one type of food I would be content with the local coconut, knowing I could always make some delicious south

Indian coconut chutney. Deep in the south of India coconut chutney is a necessary accompaniment to the fermented steamed rice cake called idli or thin crispy crepe-like dosa that millions eat every morning, but is a good accompaniment to almost any dish. This recipe combines the cooling and luxuriant oiliness of coconut with spicy and fragrant herbs, stimulating digestion and appetite.

Coconut chutney is made with whole coconut, sold intact with its brown inner husk. Choose a good coconut by shaking each one, listening for water inside. Inspect the 'eyes' of the coconut to ensure that none are broken or leaking. When you get home use a nail to puncture one of the coconut eyes that is softer than the other two. Drain the water, and if it's sweet, reserve it for later. Roast the coconut over a stove burner until the outside is a little charred and let it cool. Hold the coconut in the palm of your hand, and use the blunt end of a heavy knife to crack it open, just like you were cracking an egg. If it doesn't break, hit it again until it cracks open. Once cracked, peel the flesh away from the husk, which is made easier by roasting it before cracking. Indian grocery stores also sell hand-crank coconut grinders that can be used to remove the coconut meat from the husk without roasting it beforehand.

Ingredients
1 coconut, whole
1 tsp cumin seed
1 tsp black mustard seed
1 tsp whole black pepper
1 sprig curry leaf
1 tbsp coconut oil

Directions
Using a hand-grinder, a grater or a food processor, finely grate the fresh coconut and put aside. In a frying pan melt coconut oil and roast the cumin, mustard, black pepper and curry leaves for one minute, then add the grated coconut. Stir-fry at a medium heat for a few minutes, and add the sweet coconut water or plain water to make a paste. Simmer for 10-15 minutes, cool, and serve. For more spice add in 2-3 diced fresh green chilies, or 1-2 tsp dried red chili with the other herbs during preparation.

Coconut is an excellent food to nourish the body, skin and hair, and is used in Ayurveda to reduce inflammation and balance pitta, treat infertility and counter deficiency and vata.

Almond Milk

In a world where milk allergies and sensitivities have become increasingly prevalent, many people are turning to alternatives such as soymilk, almond milk and rice milk. Although called 'milk' none of these products have anything close to the same density of nutrients as real milk and should not be mistaken for such. In particular, I worry that milk-sensitive vegetarians will rely on dairy alternatives thinking that they provide the same level of nutrition. While I appreciate the need for milk alternatives in recipes or to flavor beverages such as tea or coffee, I can't say that I am a fan of these dairy alternatives. Most commercial products are packed in plastic-cardboard 'bricks' (e.g. 'tetra pak') which requires the beverage to be heated to relatively high temperatures when it is being filled, allowing the hot liquid to react with the polyethylene lining, likely increasing the migration of plasticizers into the beverage.[269] Other problems include the migration of chemicals from inks and dyes into the beverage.[270] Apart from packaging issues, the process of making nut milk does not adequately denature antinutrient factors (ANFs) in the legume, nut, seed or grain, making it more difficult to digest and potentially problematic for people with sensitive immune systems.

To avoid these issues I suggest making dairy alternatives at home, making sure to pasteurize them afterwards to denature the ANFs and enhance digestibility. The following recipe called for almonds but other seed or nuts can be used as well.

Ingredients
1 cup whole almonds
2-3 dates, chopped
half-stick vanilla
2-3 cardamom pods
3 cups water

Soak the almonds for 24 hours in water, drain and rinse well. Place the almonds in a blender with the chopped dates, vanilla and three times the amount of water. Blend for 3-5 minutes until smooth. Strain through a mesh strainer into a pot. Bring the liquid to a boil and then reduce to a simmer for 5 minutes. Drink warm, or store in a clean, dry vessel and allow to cool, storing covered in the refrigerator for up to 3 days. Make sure to reheat before serving.

This recipe has endless variations, and instead of almonds other nuts can be used such as hemp hearts, pumpkin seeds or sunflower seeds. Rice or oat milk is made by grinding the cereal grain to a flour, and then soaking it in water overnight. Experiment with different herbs and flavors, such as cinnamon, nutmeg, rose and lavender. Instead of date use jaggery, or after you have pasteurized and cooled the beverage, blend in a couple tablespoons of honey.

Coconut Smoothie

While I am an advocate of the big breakfast, when the weather is hot during the summer the idea of eating a large meal can be rather unappetizing. As a solution I developed a coconut smoothie my patients could eat as an alternative, and yet still give them the protein and fat boost in the morning that keeps metabolism balanced. Like many of the recipes in this book there are an endless number of variations. The base of the smoothie is coconut milk, which can be made at home by blending fresh grated coconut with a little water in a blender, and then strained. In a pinch I also recommend coconut cream concentrate or spray-dried coconut powder mixed with water, but I tend to avoid canned coconut milk due to the presence of plasticizers in the lining of the can (see p. 113).

Ingredients
1 ½ cups coconut cream
2 egg yolks, raw
1 banana
1 cup chopped fresh pineapple

Prepare the coconut cream and add it to the blender with the egg yolks, banana and pineapple. Blend until smooth, and enjoy, making sure to drink slowly. For variety try other tropical fruits such as mango or papaya, or temperate fruits such as blueberry or raspberry. You can also add in a little homemade almond milk instead of water when using a coconut cream concentrate.

Tamari Seeds

This is another macrobiotic favorite that uses the rich tangy and salty taste of Japanese soy sauce (tamari) to flavor roasted nuts. They can be eaten as a snack to take hiking or camping, or can be thrown into a veggie stir-fry at the end of cooking for added protein.

Ingredients
1 cup any shelled nuts or seeds (e.g. almond, sunflower, pumpkin, cashew)
¼ cup tamari

Directions
Soak nuts in tamari for 5 minutes, mix frequently and drain. Roast for 5-10 minutes at 250°F/120°C in the oven until lightly toasted.

Fats and Oils

Ghee

Ghee is the classic cooking fat of ancient India, used not only in a variety of both sweet and savory dishes, but also as a medicine. The term 'desi' ghee means 'home-made' ghee, and originally referred to the pure, clarified oil rendered from cultured butter. Nowadays, most commercial ghee is made from non-cultured, creamery butter, and is not made according to the traditional, time-honored methods used in Indian villages for millennia. As such, this type of clarified butter does not have the virtues and benefits of traditionally made ghee. The difference is not only in the aroma and taste of the ghee, but in its chemical composition. From an Ayurvedic perspective, ghee made from cultured butter contains within it the quality of agni, which offsets the heavy and congesting properties of regular butter and clarified butter. To make proper ghee, always make it from unsalted, cultured butter (see p. 176).

Ingredients
2 lbs (900g) unsalted cultured butter

Directions
Melt the cultured butter in ceramic, glass or stainless steel pot, either in the oven at 250°F/120°C, or on low heat on the stove. Cook for 30 minutes to one hour, until the butter separates into three distinct layers: a thin layer of impurities on the surface, the middle layer that contains the ghee, and the bottom layer which contains the milk solids. Take it off the heat and pour it off into a second bowl through a mesh strainer, leaving the congealed milk solids behind. Store the ghee in a dry glass container in a dark, cool location. To get the ghee out of the jar always use a clean dry spoon to avoid contamination and spoilage. This recipe will yield a little more than a pound (500 g) of ghee.

In Ayurveda ghee is a highly lauded food supplement, used to boost energy, improve the eyes, enhance the complexion, nourish the skin, balance the mind and nervous system, treat infertility and problems of pregnancy, counter deficiency (vata) and balance inflammation (pitta).

Tallow and Lard

While ghee is the traditional cooking fat of India, similar oils are used by other cultures in much the same way. The term tallow refers to any pure fat rendered from animal fats such as beef, bison, mutton, goose or goat, whereas the term lard exclusively refers to rendered pig fat. Regardless of the source, the technique for making tallow and lard is identical.

The key component in making tallow and lard is high quality fat, usually trimmed off the meat at the butcher. If you buy a whole or part of an animal, usually you can get the trim for free or for a small fee. Otherwise, ask your local butcher for trim taken from grass-fed, free-range meat.

Ingredients
2-3 lbs animal fat (500-1500 g)

Directions
Remove all the meat from the trim, leaving behind just the fat. Preparing tallow or lard from fat with some meat still attached may yield an off flavor in the final product. Finely chop the fat with a sharp knife, or grind it with a meat grinder or food processor, and place in a large ceramic, glass or stainless steel pot. Heat the fat in the oven at 250°F/120°C, or on low heat on the stove for 2-3 hours or more, until all the fat has been rendered. Carefully pour off the fat through a fine metal mesh strainer into a clean, dry jar and store in a cool, dry place. What's left behind is called the 'cracklings', and these are an indulgent fatty treat that can be used as a garnish in much the same way as bacon bits. This recipe will yield about 1-3 cups of rendered fat, depending on the fat content of the trim. The color should be whitish when cool, and the flavor should be fairly neutral but will vary depending on the type of animal.

Marrow fat is another excellent animal fat that has a special property to reduce vata, dryness and aging. The difference is that water is used to extract the fat from the bones to make a fatty soup stock (see p. 147). The stock is then cooled in the refrigerator or outside in cold weather so that the fat congeals on the surface of the stock. Scoop this fat off and then at low heat in a second pot, evaporate off any remaining water. Bottle in a clean dry jar, and use as a special nourishing fat to balance vata, either taken internally or applied topically.

Niter Kibbeh

Niter Kibbeh is a spiced oil traditionally used in Ethiopian and Somalian cuisine, prepared from ghee and a variety of herbs and spices. It can be used as a condiment, or as a cooking fat to add a rich flavor to savory dishes. The properties in large part depend on the herbs added, but overall, the typical herbs used for Niter Kibbeh all help to promote good digestion.

Ingredients
1 pound (450 g) ghee (p. 194)
1 head finely chopped garlic
1 thumb-sized piece of chopped fresh ginger root
½ tsp ground turmeric
½ tsp ground fenugreek seed
½ tsp ground cardamom
½ tsp ground cinnamon
¼ tsp ground nutmeg
2-3 cloves

Directions
Freshly grind herbs into a fine powder and roast in a dry pan at medium low heat for 2-3 minutes, until the aroma begins to be released. In a medium pot, melt the ghee and add the spices, garlic and ginger at low heat, and let simmer for one hour. When done, strain through a fine metal mesh strainer and store in a clean glass jar, in a cool, dry place.

Garlic Herb Oil

There are two basic ways to make a flavored oil. One method, such as Niter Kibbeh (p. 196), uses heat to render the aromatic constituents into the oil, but we can also use a more passive method called an oil infusion. Although it takes a lot longer, this kind of infused oil is ideal to preserve the delicate flavor of aromatic herbs, and helps save energy.

Oil infusions can be made with both fresh and dried herbs. If fresh herbs are used, it is best to let the plant material wilt for a couple days to reduce water content. Keeping the water content in the herbs as low as possible helps to prevent spoilage and makes for a stronger extract.

Ingredients
2 cups extra virgin olive oil
1 head coarsely chopped garlic
4 tbsp dried rosemary
2 tbsp dried basil
2 tbsp dried oregano
2 tbsp dried thyme
1 tsp crushed dried red chili

Directions
Pour olive oil into a clean dry jar, add all the herbs and seal. Set aside and give it a good shake every day for a few minutes over 2-3 weeks. Strain through a metal mesh strainer and store in a clean dry jar. Use as a condiment over steamed vegetables, or as a savory oil for low heat cooking.

According to Indian legend, garlic (lashun) originated when the devas (gods) and asuras (demons) churned the ocean of milk in heaven to render from it the elixir of life (amrita). When the elixir had been obtained, the asuras snatched it away for themselves, but then began to argue over it, and in so doing, a drop of the liquid spilt from the cup. The drop fell from heaven and landed on earth, and from this drop the garlic plant grew. It is thus said that garlic has all the benefits of the elixir of life, but because it arose from trickery and dispute that garlic can also inflame the passions and aggravate pitta. In herbal medicine garlic is a powerful antimicrobial herb used in bacterial and fungal infections, and is also used to counter deficiency, promote fertility, enhance digestion, boost the immune system and alleviate cough.

Snacks, Sweets and Libations

Mango Chat

The Indian word for snack is 'chat', and rather than a particular kind of food, instead refers to a diverse array of foods all flavored with a spicy mixture called 'chat masala'. Among the different foods traditionally prepared with chat are fruits such as mango, papaya and melon, but I use just about any fruit including peach, pear and apple. According to Ayurveda, most sweet fruits have a cooling quality, and although deliciously refreshing can be congesting and cloying, promoting excess mucus and water retention. Chat masala is added to the fresh fruit to provide a salty and pungent flavor that balances the sweetness, making the fruit easier to digest.

There are a huge number of chat varieties that all make use of familiar Indian spices such as cumin and black pepper. What makes chat unique however, is its use of sour flavored herbs such as amchur (unripe mango powder) and anardana (pomegranate seed powder). Where these more exotic herbs aren't available, fresh squeezed lime can be used instead.

Ingredients
3 large mangos, not quite fully ripened
2 tsp coriander seed powder
2 tsp cumin seed powder
1 tsp amchar (mango seed powder)
½ tsp ajwain seed powder
¼ tsp cayenne powder
¼ tsp hing powder
1-2 tsp pink salt
1 tbsp extra-virgin walnut, hazelnut or hemp oil

Directions
Wash mangos, peel and cut away from the large pit in the middle. Chop mango into half-inch chunks and place into a bowl. In a separate pan at medium-low heat, roast the hing powder for 30 seconds, and then add the remaining herbs and salt, cooking for another half-minute. Sprinkle over top the

mango, add the oil and toss together. Garnish with fresh mint or cilantro. Serves four or more people.

Blood Building Syrup

All systems of traditional medicine make extensive use of the medicinal properties of both fresh and dried fruit, cooked with water to make a compote, or prepared as medicinal jams and syrups. Ayurveda maintains a large class of medicinal jams called lehyas, which means 'to lick', referring to the method of administration. While they aren't exactly like deserts, compotes, jams and syrups are a very pleasant to get the medicine down, and are particularly suited to both vata and pitta conditions. The following 'Blood Building Syrup' is an excellent preparation to help build up the blood in anemia, infertility, exhaustion, and immunodeficiency, or when recovering from chronic disease, medical treatments (e.g. chemotherapy) or surgery. Although it is prepared as a syrup in this recipe, to prepare as a compote simply stew the fruit with the herbs and serve it without processing it further.

Ingredients
½ cup chopped dried figs
½ cup dried goji berries
½ cup dried prunes
½ cup Chinese red dates
1 oz shatavari root (tien men dong or asparagus root)
1 oz cured rehmannia (shu di huang)
1 oz astragalus root (huang qi)
1 oz American ginseng (xi yang shen)
2 quarts (liters) water
2-3 tbsp ghee
2 tbsp pippali powder
1 tsp cardamom powder
1 tsp cinnamon powder
½ tsp clove powder
¼ tsp pink salt
1 cup organic molasses (approximately)

Add the dried fruit and herbs (shatavari, rehmannia, astragalus, American ginseng) into a pot along with 2 quarts of water, bring to a boil and simmer until it is reduced to a syrup-like consistency and the fruit and herbs are squishy (about 1 hour). Allow the fruit-herb decoction to cool and then mix in a blender until smooth. Strain the liquid through a mesh strainer into a measuring cup, taking note of exactly how much liquid you are left with. In a separate pan, melt the ghee on medium heat and add the pippali, cardamom, cinnamon, clove and pink salt. Cook for a minute and then add the fruit-herb decoction to this, along with an equal part molasses. Cook on low heat for about 10-15 minutes, stirring frequently. Pour into a clean, dry glass bottle, seal and store in a cool location. Dose is 1-2 tbsp twice daily, with warm water.

Quinoa Cake

This recipe is the only borrowed recipe in this book, and it comes from a family member who is a food lover and knows what it's like to suffer because of it. Made with quinoa, this cake recipe is so delectable and moist that it far exceeds any expectation you might have of regular cake. Although I might be hard pressed to call this a 'medicinal' food, it does contain over a cup of organic cocoa powder, and in my considered opinion, chocolate is both a medicine and a food – so enjoy and be happy. This would be a nice weekly dessert for a regular Sunday dinner.

Ingredients
¾ cup quinoa (fermented, p. 126)
1 ½ cups water
¾ cup butter
¼ - ½ cup milk (or almond milk, or water)
4 large eggs
1 tsp vanilla
1 cup jaggery (gur)
1 cup cocoa powder
1 ½ tsp aluminum-free baking powder
½ tsp baking soda
salt

Directions

Drain soaked quinoa, rinse, bring to a boil in twice the volume of water and let simmer for 20 minutes. Allow to cool, fluff with a fork. Melt the butter and set aside to cool, greasing two 8-inch round baking pans and preheating the oven to 350 F. In a blender combine the milk, eggs, vanilla and cooked quinoa, and blend to a custard-like consistency. In a separate bowl whisk together the jaggery, cocoa powder, baking powder, baking soda and a pinch of salt. Mix well then add the wet ingredients to the dry, mix well, and then pour into two cake pans. Bake for 40-45 minutes or until a knife comes out clean. Serve with fresh whipped cream sweetened with a little maple syrup, or homemade strawberry-rose ice cream.

Parvati's Delight

This sweet is named after the goddess of beauty and desire, a voluptuous Indian Aphrodite wedded to her Lord Shiva, himself represented by a giant lingam, or phallus. As the name suggests, this is meant to be an aphrodisiac food, but is also just a very pleasant dessert, perhaps with a little red wine after dinner for an intimate moment. The recipe has endless variations, depending on your desire.

Ingredients
6 oz (squares) of unsweetened chocolate
½ cup honey
¼ cup tahini
2-3 tbsp maca powder
2 tbsp. clarified butter
2 tbsp ashwagandha powder, finely sieved
2 tbsp shatavari (tien men dong), finely sieved
1 tsp cinnamon powder, finely sieved
1 tsp cardamom powder, finely sieved
1 tsp nutmeg powder, finely sieved
1 tsp clove powder, finely sieved
1 tsp black pepper powder, finely sieved
rice or coconut flour, as needed

Melt chocolate and clarified butter together. Add powders of maca, ashwagandha, shatavari, cinnamon, cardamom, nutmeg, clove and black pepper. Mix into the chocolate/ghee combination and simmer over a low heat for 10 minutes. Cool in pan until warm. Pour over honey in a separate bowl and mix well. Add tahini and mix into a dough, adding in a little rice or coconut flour if it seems too wet. Roll into half-inch sized balls and place on a plate in the freezer to cool. When it's ready, roll the balls in some icing sugar, cocoa powder or licorice root powder. Keep cool, and enjoy. Dose is 2-4 chocolates, or more, depending on your plans for the evening...

Burgundy Bitters

Alcohol is an effective solvent for many of the active constituents found in medicinal plants, but some types of alcohol such as wine contain too low a percentage of alcohol to be all that efficient. The low percent alcohol in wine is also insufficient to preserve shelf life and prevent it from being fermented by lactic acid bacteria and turning it into vinegar. To enhance the extractive properties of wine as well as to preserve shelf life, any wine can be fortified with distilled liquor, such as brandy, whiskey, vodka or rum. Common fortified wines include port, sherry, madeira, marsala and vermouth.

Generally speaking, fortified wines can be broadly classified into either apéritifs, taken before meals to enhance the appetite, or digestifs, which are taken after meals to promote good digestion. Apéritifs are usually made with bitter herbs, which stimulate bile synthesis in the liver, whereas digestifs are made with aromatic and spicy herbs that promote good digestion and alleviate gas and bloating. Although separated into different categories, it is possible to make a fortified wine that contains both these properties, making it suitable for before or after meals, such as this recipe for Burgundy Bitters:

Ingredients
2 tbsp crushed gentian root
1 tbsp crushed anise seed
1 tbsp coriander seed
1 tbsp crushed dried ginger root

1 tbsp dried orange peel
375 mL burgundy wine
375 mL brandy
½ cup honey, or as desired

Directions

Mix wine and brandy together in a mason jar, and add in the honey and herbs. Seal and give a good shake for a few minutes. Let this sit for two weeks, giving it a good shake every couple of days. Strain, decant and filter. Dose is one sherry glass, before or after supper.

There are a huge number of variations on this theme, depending on the herbs and the amount of honey or sweetener used. Other herbs to consider include exotic herbs such as cinnamon, fennel, nutmeg, cardamom, mace and clove, or more European herbs such as marjoram, chamomile, poppy seed and juniper. Some recipes call for bitters such as wormwood (*Artemisia absinthium*), a potent herb that has anti-parasite effects as well as mild psychoactive properties. In South America, alcoholic preparations are often made from damiana (*Turnera diffusa*), a bitter-tasting herb that has aphrodisiac and sexual restorative properties. In China, fortified wines are frequently made from restorative herbs such as dang gui, Chinese ginseng and astragalus. And instead of honey, experiment with other sweeteners such as molasses, maple syrup, treacle or jaggery.

Hot Toddy

It was an irresistible compulsion that caused me to include this recipe, not just because it's my namesake, but because hot toddy has a universally good reputation as a remedy for colds. From the perspective of Ayurveda, distilled liquor is pungent in flavor, and has a hot and dry energy that is useful for overcoming congestion. Originally based on the fermented palm sap drink called 'todi', the name became attached to a Scottish drink made from whiskey and aromatic herbs, served warm.

Ingredients
½ oz whiskey or rum
1 cinnamon stick, broken into pieces
2 cloves, crushed
2 cardamom pods, crushed
3-4 slices of ginger
¼ tsp fresh grated nutmeg
1 cup water
1 tbsp jaggery (cane sugar)
1 tsp fresh lemon juice

Directions
Crush cloves and cardamom with the cinnamon stick in a mortar and pestle. Bring water to boil in a pot and add in the cinnamon, cloves, ginger and nutmeg, reduce to a simmer, and cook for 10 minutes uncovered. Add one ounce whiskey or rum, stirring in the sugar and lemon. Strain into a cup and serve with a cinnamon stick. Take one cup in the evening to relieve congestion and promote a sound sleep. For symptoms of dryness mix in 1 tsp of cultured butter.

Section Four: Detoxification

What is Detoxification?

Among the more popular but nonetheless controversial topics both within and without the field of natural healing is the concept of detoxification. Whereas advocates swear by detoxification as a kind of panacea, skeptics dismiss it as fanciful nonsense. In part both are right, and both are wrong – and I shall explain why.

Detoxification is a precise scientific term that is most often used in the context of toxicology, a branch of medical science concerned with the study and removal of external toxins such as heavy metals, drugs and alcohol. More broadly however, detoxification is an inherent element of physiological function that is built into every cell of the body, attending not only to the biotransformation of poisons, but also to internal toxins that naturally accumulate through normal metabolic processes. Although discrete biological factors are at play in each separate process, the basic nature of what is meant by detoxification is nonetheless the same – the rendering of actively toxic compounds into relatively inert ones, regardless of their origin. Once these compounds are biotransformed they can be easily removed from the body, dumped from the tissues into the lymph and blood, and from there into the mucus, sweat, urine, bile and feces for elimination.

Detoxification is a crucial element in the maintenance of homeostasis, an optimal physiological environment in which there is a free flow of nutrients into cells while wastes are discharged from the body with little interruption. No biologist or medical doctor would ever argue with detoxification as a biological fact, and few would argue that it is a crucial component of good health. It should be clear that alterations to patterns in the way each of us detoxifies various substances can have a dramatic impact upon our health, and especially how we might respond to certain medical treatments. For example, it is well established that citrus fruits like grapefruit alter detoxification pathways in the liver, inhibiting enzymes (CYP 3A4) that detoxify certain drugs, leading to an increase in the bioavailability of these drugs and possible overdose.[271] In contrast, herbs such as St. John's wort (*Hypericum perforatum*) enhance the activity of these same enzymes, promoting the excretion of certain drugs and thus decreasing their effectiveness in the body.[272]

Detoxification in the context of maintaining good health, or homeostasis, is exactly what is intended by the concept of detoxification in the natural health industry. The problem lies not with the concept, which has a basis in both good science and tradition, but with the profligate proliferation of cleansing and detoxification products that have less to do with cleansing your body than they do with cleansing you of your cash and credit. Many of these products are ridiculously over-priced with very little in the way of support except for the most rudimentary of concepts reduced to the bland pandering of marketing noise. The packaging is wasteful, the quality of ingredients is only sometimes "organic", and many of the claims made for these products skirt the edge of reality. Although not exactly illegal many of these products are shamelessly unethical. And when this is the criticism that is raised by skeptics, I wholly agree with them.

As in science, detoxification is a concept that is well represented in traditional societies all over the world. Even what we might call primitive peoples understood well the delicate balance of health, and over generations of practice developed methods to enhance detoxification pathways in the body, such as by fasting and sweating. The basic premise behind these practices is that internally produced toxins are produced all the time and accumulate very easily, and that in order to maintain this delicate balance of health we can assist the processes of physical detoxification. Traditional peoples recognize many occasions when detoxification processes are naturally impaired, such as in poor weather, with an inappropriate diet or during great emotional stress. On the balance there are many so many opportunities for detoxification pathways to be overwhelmed that regular detoxification is not only helpful, but a necessary component of good health.

Origin of wastes and toxins

In all systems of traditional medicine, as in Ayurveda, a poorly functioning digestive system is a key component in the production of **wastes and toxins** (ama, lit. 'undigested food').

Ingested foods that are not broken down properly due to deficient or otherwise impaired digestive functions alter the bowel ecology, cause direct damage to the gut wall, add to the toxic burden of the liver, and promote immune dysfunction. While skeptics might find this time-honored notion naïve, scientific research is beginning to validate this complex relationship between diet, digestion and chronic disease.[273, 274, 275, 276] It is for these reasons that herbalists all over the world consider digestion to be the root of health.

In addition to poor digestion, toxins accumulate and disrupt normal physiological activities when the eliminatory faculties of the body are impaired. According to the Western herbal tradition there are five basic **eliminatory faculties**: the kidneys, liver, bowel, lungs and skin. The eliminatory mechanisms represented by each one of these organ systems function in a synergistic fashion, each according to their innate capacity, to process and remove toxins from the body. When any one of these eliminatory systems is impaired in some way the net result is that the toxic burden must be taken on by other organ systems, decreasing their functional efficiency. Thus when bowel or kidney function is impaired, the result might be an increase in respiratory mucus or skin eruptions. Observing and integrating these relationships between the organs of elimination is a key element of traditional medicine.

Apart from the toxins that accumulate through poor digestion and faulty elimination, it is clear that toxins can come from other sources including the environment and our lifestyle. One of the hallmarks of modernity is that we are exposed to an enormous number of pollutants, from chemicals like pesticides and heavy metals, to energy like ionizing radiation and electromagnetism. These all add to the toxic burden of the body, weakening tissues and organs and impairing the eliminative mechanisms we need to stay healthy. Another source are pathogens such as fungi and bacteria that invade and replicate in the body, often when the vital function of the body is obstructed, creating toxins that impair cellular functions and promote toxicity. Even chronic stress, experienced by so many in our modern hectic life, has the capacity to disrupt this delicate balance of nutrition and elimination.

Signs and symptoms of toxicity

While we are all naturally a little bit toxic, when the toxins build up they overwhelm digestion and the body's eliminative faculties. According to Ayurveda, the presence or absence of toxins yields characteristic signs and symptoms:

Presence of toxins	Absence of toxins
Circulatory congestion, cold body	Circulation normal, warm body
Loss of strength, heaviness of body	Normal strength, lightness of body
Lethargy and fatigue after eating	Energized and revitalized after eating
Poor appetite	Good appetite
Indigestion	Good digestion
Constipation	At least two bowel movements daily
Sinking stools with mucus congestion	Normal stools (brown, floating)
Increased urination	Normal urination
Joint swelling, pain or inflammation	Absence of joint swelling, pain or inflammation
Headache	No headache
Thick tongue coating	Clear or thin white coating
Puffy eyes, dull, lacking luster; poor vision	Absence of puffiness, eyes bright and shining; good vision
Symptoms worse with cold and damp weather or climates	Health unaffected by changes in weather or climate

Methods of Detoxification

There are many ways to detoxify the body, from making simple alterations to one's diet, to fasting on nothing except water. The key component however is the decreased consumption of food, altering the metabolic balance so that you are expending at least as much energy as you are ingesting. The more dramatically we tip the metabolic balance towards energy expenditure the more efficient the process – but only to a point, and then it becomes counter-productive. Detoxification by its very nature is part of the rest and restorative system of the body and cannot occur when the body is under stress. This means that overdoing it, or trying to detox while following your regular daily regimen, isn't the best idea. The proper approach to detoxification requires that you reduce your activity levels significantly, while simultaneously reducing your nutrient intake. Going to the cottage, to a retreat, or just taking some time off work or from the family, are all good opportunities for detoxification.

Fasting

Fasting is an important component of a cleansing and detoxification regimen, and many different forms exist, depending on the person, the nature of their health, and other factors such as the season and climate. There are several different kinds of fasts or cleanses, and they can be broken down into three basic regimens including water fasting (p. 215), juice fasting (p. 216) and a simple diet (p. 219).

When we eat, the food is digested into a slurry of nutrients gathered from the digestive tract and carried to the liver via the hepatic portal vein. The liver then takes these nutrients and generates them into the various components that form the bodily tissues, listening, measuring and then deciding which kind and how much of each particular nutrient needs to be generated. At the same time, the liver receives all of the normal metabolic wastes of the body, either recycling these for further use, or dumping them into the bile for elimination. Along with the liver, the kidneys play a key role in deciding what components of the blood need to be rendered and eliminated, and which to keep and recycle.

When our diet is proper and we are in good health there is an optimal balance between the nutrients we consume, how they are processed, and what is eliminated. When our diet is poor and the food isn't properly digested, it increases the workload of the liver and creates a kind of backlog in the body. Normal metabolic wastes that should be eliminated become trapped, impairing homeostatic mechanisms, weakening and damaging tissues, promoting aging and disease.

Fasting is an important method to alleviate this metabolic backlog, taking the burden of processing nutrients off the liver and kidneys, allowing them to focus on the elimination of wastes. Reducing the intake of food, or at least the complexity of the diet, creates more 'space' for the liver, kidneys and other eliminative organs to function.

Candidates and criteria for fasting

Generally speaking, an intensive fast should only be undertaken by a person that is in good health. In some cases certain types of fasts can be recommended for the infirm or elderly, but there will never be a complete abstention from food. Similarly, children and pregnant women should avoid fasts except for a simple diet, and even then, only for a limited period of time. During a fast the living space should be free of too many distractions, and it is best if the person could avoid working or studying during this period. Ideally, a fast should be a time of free expression and spiritual investigation, which is very much in harmony with the physiological process of detoxification. When the body is tense and the mind is stressed, wastes and toxins are much more difficult to remove. The effect of each type fast and its impact on the doshas is reviewed on page 221.

Timing a fast

A fast should follow a seasonal pattern, undertaken between the juncture of winter and spring to reduce kapha and pitta, and between summer and fall to reduce vata and pitta. The period of time between fall and winter is when the body focuses on building up and storing energy, protecting itself like a plant extending its roots deep in the soil. Fasting in winter runs counter to the physiological effects of the season.

Preparing for a fast

Regardless of the method of fasting some measure of preparation is required before beginning a detoxification regimen. If you are drink alcohol, smoke or drink a lot of coffee or tea, it's a good idea to wean these items out of the diet before going on the fast. Indulging in them while fasting corrupts the whole purpose of going on fast in the first place. If you take prescription drugs it's a good idea to review them to see if they should be taken with food, and to carefully review potential drug interactions with your health care practitioner. If you are diabetic then water or juice fasting is not the best approach to cleansing, and you are better off eating a low-carb diet with lots of non-starchy vegetables. If you feel that you are particularly toxic, work your way into the fast slowly, consuming only raw fruits and vegetables the first day, a complete water fast for the next 2-3 days, followed by a juice fast over the next 4-6 days. In weaker people or in vata conditions, fast on simple foods such as kitchari for 7-14 days, followed by a 2-3 day juice fast, and then another 7-14 day fast on simple foods.

Fasting on water

Water fasting is an intensive method of fasting that is only indicated for excess weight (kapha) or inflammation (pitta), and is contraindicated in any kind of deficiency (vata). During a water fast the body is spared any nutrients, and will essentially begin to eat itself, breaking down muscle glycogen into blood sugar, and then when this is consumed, breaking down fatty acids stored in adipose tissues, turning them into ketones. Water fasting will often promote immediate weight loss, sometimes very rapidly, and should not be followed for more than 2-3 days. If someone wishes to fast on water for longer, such as a week or more, they should be under proper supervision, or at the very least, be regularly monitored by friends and family. One of the effects of using ketones as energy is that they can make the blood more acidic. **Danger signs** include a fruity odor of acetone on the breath, mental confusion, extreme lethargy, difficulty breathing, nausea, vomiting, and dryness of the skin and mucus membranes. One way to prevent against these effects is to consume an abundance of alkalizing fluids such as soup stock (p. 147) and teas made with mineral-rich herbs including nettle, dandelion leaf and oatstraw. Distilled water is sometimes recommended for water fasting, but due to the lack of dissolved solutes can easily disrupt the delicate electrolyte balance of the body, and is not recommended for more than 2-3 days in a row.

Fasting on juice

Juice fasting combines the benefits of water fasting with the introduction of alkalizing substances that help to buffer the blood against acidosis. Further, juice fasting provides somewhat of a psychological buffer, since something of substance is being consumed. Juice fasting can also protect against low blood sugar (hypoglycemia), but if the juices are consumed to excess or consumed too quickly, they can promote transient states of high blood sugar (hyperglycemia), which can rebound into low blood sugar (hypoglycemia). The best way to avoid this is to dilute the juice by half with water, and consume it over a longer period of time, such as a quart of juice slowly sipped over an hour. As saying goes, "drink your food, and chew your juice." Chewing the juice by swishing it around in the mouth ensures that it undergoes some initial digestion in the upper gastrointestinal tract.

Generally speaking, juice fasting has a good effect on all three doshas, but can be employed to a different extent and with different types of juice for each dosha. Fruits and vegetables with a sweet, sour, salty and mildly pungent flavor are better for vata (deficiency), whereas a combination of sweet, bitter and astringent tastes are better for pitta (inflammation). For kapha (mucus), the taste of the juice should be more bitter, astringent and pungent, although the base of the juice should still be a little sweet, just to provide some food energy.

Vata-reducing juices
Vata-reducing juice targets about 70% sweet-tasting fruits and vegetables, 15% salty, 15% sour. Add in a small amount of a

pungent herb, such as ginger or basil, and salts such as sea salt or saindhava. Examples include:

- Sweet fruits: apple, raspberry, blueberry, grape, açaí, guava, passionfruit
- Sour fruits: orange, kiwi, strawberry, grapefruit, lime
- Sweet vegetables: carrot, beet, cucumber, winter melon
- Salty vegetables: celery, garlic, dill, savory
- Pungent herbs: ginger, cilantro, basil, parsley

Pitta-reducing juices

Pitta-reducing juice targets about 70% sweet-tasting fruits and vegetables, 30% bitter and astringent vegetables, only ever with a hint of ginger to prevent any indigestion. Examples include:

- Sweet fruits: apple, raspberry, blueberry, grape, açaí, guava, passionfruit
- Sweet vegetables: carrot, beet, cucumber, winter melon
- Bitter and astringent vegetables and herbs: celery tops, lettuce, cabbage, chard, kale, bitter melon, endive, fresh turmeric root, cilantro, parsley

Kapha-reducing juices

Kapha-reducing juice targets about 50% sweet-tasting vegetables, 40% bitter and astringent vegetables, and 10% pungent flavors. Examples include:

- Sweet vegetables: carrot, beet, cucumber, winter melon
- Bitter fruits: lemon, lime
- Bitter and astringent vegetables: mustard greens, beet greens, bitter melon, celery tops, lettuce, cabbage, chard, kale, zucchini
- Pungent herbs: ginger, fresh turmeric, cilantro, parsley

Beyond basing the choice of juice ingredients on the way the flavors affect each dosha, we can also compare the general properties of each food, and its effect in the body. **Tart fruits** such as raspberry, blueberry, strawberry, guava and passionfruit have cooling, anti-inflammatory properties, and are particularly good for improving the health of the circulatory system, in diseases of the eyes, cardiovascular disease, varicose veins and diabetes. **Acid fruits** like lemon, lime, and grapefruit all help to sharpen the appetite and enhance metabolism. **Carrots** are particularly good for the eyes and skin, and gently detoxify the body. **Beets** are great for the liver, gall bladder and bowel. **Cucumber** restores the basic watery constitution of the body, helping to reduce heat and moisturize the body. **Winter melon** has a cooling energy and helps to nourish and balance the mind. Leafy greens such as **chard**, **kale**, **cabbage**, and **broccoli** alkalize the blood and enhance liver metabolism, and are the most cleansing and detoxifying juices to consume, helping mobilize deep-seated toxins such as pesticides and heavy metals. **Mustard greens** alkalize and purify the blood, as well as open up and stimulate the bodily channels for elimination. Leafy herbs like **cilantro**, **parsley** and **basil** share the properties of leafy greens, but also to sharpen the digestion, dispel gas and colic, and enhance circulation. Fresh **ginger** is an excellent herb to promote good circulation, reduce mucus, as well as prevent any griping caused by the harder to digest components of leafy greens. **Bitter melon** (karela) is another useful detoxifying vegetable, used in smaller amounts to enhance liver function, promote elimination, and balance blood sugar levels. Fresh **turmeric** root is also good to support liver function, reduce inflammation and inhibit joint and muscle pain.

Breaking a water or juice fast

On the morning of breaking the fast consume, solid fruits and vegetables along with the juice, followed by an evening meal of a clear meat or vegetable broth with steamed vegetables. The following day, breakfast again should be comprised of solid fruits or vegetables, as well as juice, followed by a small, normal lunch and supper. By the third day a normal dietary pattern can be implemented. To keep the spirit of the fast, a one day biweekly juice fast is an excellent strategy to maintain health. In traditional cultures this type of fasting was often marked by religious holidays, such as on the day of the full and new moon of each lunar cycle.

Fasting on a simple diet

Another form of fasting is to consume a **simple diet** over an extended period of time. Unlike water and juice fasting, this method is better for individuals who are weakened by disease or age, in both children and adults. It is the best approach for those suffering from vata conditions and also anyone under any kind of chronic stress, such as work, family or school. Eating a simple diet avoids the consumption of complex foods or potentially problematic food combinations that can play havoc with digestion and promote the creation of toxins.

Fruit diet

A fast on nothing but fruit is probably the simplest form of this diet, but should only be undertaken when the weather is warm and the fruit is locally available (p. 43). In tropical countries, fruit such as papaya, coconut, mango, guava, melon, passionfruit and grape are all good choices, whereas in temperate climates fruit such as apple, raspberry and blueberry are more suitable. The fruit should be chewed slowly to ensure proper digestion, prepared with herbs and spices (p. 198), and taken as 3-5 small meals throughout the day.

Certain fruits such as grape are reputed to be very helpful to treat serious diseases and can be consumed as the sole food for several weeks, up to 40 days. A fruitarian diet however should not be undertaken for any longer than this, and is contraindicated in hypoglycemia and diabetes. From a strictly Ayurvedic perspective, a fruit diet is an excellent choice for reducing pitta, but because fruit is cooling in nature a fruitarian diet may be contraindicated in vata and kapha conditions.

Vegetable diet

Another variation on the simple diet is to eat nothing except steamed vegetables including starchy root vegetables such as sweet potatoes, squash, rutabaga and beet, along with an equal volume of leafy green vegetables. Raw vegetables are avoided on this kind of diet, and care should be taken to properly cook the starchy vegetables so that they soft and digestible, but not overcook the greens. Small amounts of fats such as coconut, butter and olive oil can be eaten with the vegetables, as well as with a little sea salt, pepper and other aromatic spices to enhance digestion. If digestion is weak these vegetables can be as a prepared in a soup stock (p. 147). This simple vegetable diet helps to balance all three doshas, and can be easily modified to address specific imbalances. For example, if kapha is imbalanced, reduce the fat and starch component and add more spicy herbs such as cayenne, black pepper, garlic, and ginger. To balance pitta, use only a little fat, and emphasize cooling spices such as coriander, turmeric, mint and fennel. For vata, use a little more fat (if well-tolerated), and emphasize vegetables prepared in broth, with mild herbs such as cumin, ginger, ajwain and pink salt.

Grains and legumes

Another variation on the concept of a simple diet is to simply eat a diet of cereals and legumes, ideally, prepared in a soup (p. 147) to enhance digestion. In Ayurveda, the most common recipe is 'kitchari', a simple food prepared from mung beans, rice, and spices (p. 180). Soupy grains or kitchari can be consumed over an extended period of time, for each meal of the day, for a minimum of 12 days to as long as several months. Although not necessarily an optimal source of nutrients, kitchari does provide the body sufficient protein, fat and carbohydrate to maintain the body in a good state of health. One variation is to add steamed vegetables to help with detoxification and supply the body with additional nutrients. This forms a good basis for a vegetarian diet, along with dairy products such as boiled milk (p. 173), yogurt (p. 174) and ghee (p. 194).

Effects of fasting

Some of the initial symptoms that can occur during the first few days of fasting include headache, temperature sensitivity, fatigue, and irritability. There may be withdrawal symptoms, such as a craving for sugar, bread or milk, which may be indicative of addictive food allergies. Likewise, there may be a craving for other addictive substances, like tobacco, alcohol, chocolate, or marijuana. After this initial period there is usually a release of creative energy, and especially with water or juice fasting, many people experience visions, either in dream or through poetry, painting and music. Among the other symptoms that can occur during a fast are bad breath, pimples, oily hair and skin, an increase in urination, and increased earwax and mucus production. Sometimes there may be aches and pains, especially in joints that were previously injured but have now healed. This is an example of Herring's Law, that as rejuvenation occurs, ailments and symptoms never completely resolved resurface in a transient fashion. From the perspective of Ayurveda, fasting and detoxification is all about peeling away layers of negative influences that mask our true constitution, and who we really are.

Choosing a fast

It is important to properly discriminate between the different types of fasts, when to implement them and what type of people are more suited to the different methods. Implementing a fasting regimen based on the observance of the doshas is one useful way to do this:

Method	Vata	Pitta	Kapha
Water-fasting (p. 215)	Increases vata; avoid	Balances pitta; one week max.	Decreases kapha; two weeks max.
Juice-fasting (p. 216)	Balances vata; one week max. Emphasize vata reducing juices	Balances pitta; two weeks max. Emphasize pitta reducing juices	Balances kapha; four weeks max. Emphasize kapha reducing juices
Simple diet (p. 219)	Balances vata; one month max. Emphasize meat soup, vegetables, kitchari.	Balances pitta; three months max. Emphasize fruit, vegetables, kitchari, khadi.	Balances kapha; six months max. Emphasize dhal, vegetables, kitchari; avoid fruit.

Herbs and Detoxification

The plant world abounds with helpful allies, and especially those that help to remove toxins and restore good health. Imagine the air in the busy downtown core of any city, and now contrast this to the crisp, delightful fragrance of a rainforest. It doesn't take a biology degree to understand that plants clean and purify the environment, and now even government and industry are getting into the act: planting gingko trees along polluted urban avenues to clean the air, and using vetiver grass in the bioremediation of industrial sites. The only difference is that herbalists extend this effect to the body, and the internal use of medicinal plants: but it is exactly the same principle.

Traditional methods of detoxification involve the upregulation and support of the eliminative faculties of the body, including the liver, bowel, skin, kidneys and lungs. Through careful observation over thousands of years of practice, herbalists have been able to identify which herbs affect these systems. From a scientific perspective, herbal medicines often exert their effects by modifying elements of cellular function such as gene expression. In this way, an herb that influences a particular organ also targets that element of cellular function, and thus when we are 'cleansing the liver', the actual effect may be on organelles such as the endoplasmic reticulum, which packages and processes wastes for elimination on a cellular level. In this way, herbalists are conducting a rather sophisticated form of gene therapy, and one that is attracting a growing number of scientific researchers.[277]

Digestive herbs

According to Ayurveda, before undertaking any measure of detoxification the body must first be prepared by enhancing the digestive fire. This is called **ama-pachana,** or 'toxin-cooking', in which the digestive fire is stoked to help to clear out wastes and 'burn' any residues in the system. In turn, this allows for the digestive tract to receive other wastes liberated from deeper tissues in the body, which through the process of detoxification will gradually be displaced to the digestive tract for elimination. While ama-pachana is often undertaken as a separate approach in Ayurveda, it can also be included as part of an ongoing herbal therapy to promote detoxification, along with a simple diet, or during fasting. Useful herbs to stoke the digestive fire are a class of herbs called **stimulants**, which regulate appetite, enhance circulation and remove congestion:

- cayenne fruit *(Capsicum spp.)*
- cinnamon bark *(Cinnamomum zeylanicum)*
- bayberry bark *(Myrica cerifera)*
- black pepper fruit *(Piper nigrum)*
- prickly ash berry *(Zanthoxylum americanum)*
- ginger root *(Zingiber officinalis)*

Similar to stimulants are the **carminatives**: herbs that contain fragrant volatile constituents that enhance digestive activity by reducing spasm and drying excessive dampness. Although these herbs are warming they are not nearly so strong as stimulants, and have a specific application in poor motility, bloating and flatulence. Some of these herbs, and especially the mints, also have an ascending energy and are thus contraindicated in heartburn:

- dill seed *(Anethum graveolens)*
- orange peel *(Citrus reticulata)*
- musta rhizome *(Cyperus rotundus)*
- cardamom seed *(Elettaria cardamomum)*
- fennel seed *(Foeniculum vulgare)*
- shan zha berry *(Crataegus pinnatifida)*

Some herbs appear to contain constituents that resemble the body's own digestive enzymes, such as the protein-digestimg enzyme papain in papaya leaf *(Carica papaya)*, or the starch-digesting enzyme amylase in rice sprouts *(Oryza sativa)*.

Cholagogues
Perhaps the most useful group of herbs for detoxification are the bitter-tasting herbs which upregulate bile synthesis and excretion in the liver – the body's primary organ of detoxification. Called **cholagogues**, or 'bile stimulants', the bitter taste of these herbs stimulates a cascade of hormones stimulated by taste receptors on the tongue, resulting in increased liver

activity. Many of these herbs are also called **alteratives**, which refers to a property by which the blood is purified of its toxic burden. Cholagogues are a vital part of any detoxification protocol, and sometimes form the entire therapeutic basis of detoxification. Important cholagogues include:

- dandelion root *(Taraxacum officinalis)*
- barberry root *(Berberis vulgaris)*
- buplerum root *(Bupleurum falcatum)*
- turmeric root *(Curcuma longa)*
- huang qin root *(Scutellaria baicalensis)*
- fringetree root *(Chionanthus virginica)*

Alteratives

Alteratives are herbs that have a beneficial effect upon the blood, primarily through their influence upon the lymphatic system and liver, stimulating glandular secretion and improving assimilation and nutrition. Many but not all have a bitter taste and are also cholagogues. Examples of alteratives include:

- garlic bulb *(Allium sativum)*
- burdock root *(Arctium lappa)*
- cleavers herb *(Galium aparine)*
- red clover blossoms *(Trifolium pratense)*
- nettle herb *(Urtica dioica)*
- poke root *(Phytolacca decandra)*

Aperients

Aperients are herbs that have a direct activity upon the elimination of toxins in the body by gently stimulating the large bowel. Although it's the liver's job to process and dump wastes into the bile, it is the bowel's job to eliminate this via the feces. Alterations and especially inefficiencies in bowel function lead to increased transit time, and the greater potential for these toxins to be reabsorbed by the intestinal mucosa and into the blood stream. Including aperients in a formula ensures that the wastes processed by the liver are being properly discharged from the bowel. Examples of aperient herbs include:

- cascara sagrada bark *(Rhamnus purshiana)*
- butternut bark *(Juglans cinerea)*
- rhubarb root *(Rheum palmatum)*
- senna pod *(Cassia angustifolia)*
- haritaki fruit *(Terminalia chebula)*
- trivrit *(Operculina turpethum)*

Diuretics and diaphoretics

Diuretics and diaphoretics are herbs that act upon the elimination of liquid wastes in the body, either through the stimulation of sweat (diaphoresis) or urine (diuresis). Typically, diuretic herbs are taken cold or at room temperature, and diaphoretic herbs are taken warm. This class of herbs is nowhere near as powerful as pharmacological diuretics, at least not in their potential to cause serious side effects or disrupt electrolyte balance. Many of these herbs can also have a hypotensive effect and are used therapeutically to reduce water retention, as well as treat urinary tract infection.

- yarrow herb *(Achillea millefolium)*
- couch grass herb *(Agropyron repens)*
- parsley herb *(Petroselinum crispum)*
- pipsissewa herb *(Chimaphila umbellata)*
- dandelion leaf *(Taraxacum officinalis)*
- gokshura seed *(Tribulus terrestris)*

Expectorants and mucolytics

Expectorants and mucolytics are a class of herbs that help to dispel excess mucus from the respiratory system. In many cases this effect is also exhibited by herbs that act on digestion, but for the purpose of detoxification specific attention should also be given to the lungs . Many of these herbs are spicy or astringent in action, helping to warm the lungs, thin the mucus and restore tone to the mucus membranes. Examples of expectorants include:

- mullein leaf *(Verbascum thapsus)*
- vasa leaf *(Adhatoda vasica)*
- elecampane root *(Inula helenium)*
- tulsi leaf *(Ocimum sanctum)*
- bibhitaki fruit *(Terminalia chebula)*

- true fir bark *(Abies grandis)*

Putting it all together

The basis of any herbal formula to promote detoxification should be carefully matched with the signs and symptoms of a patient. If for example the liver is diseased, then care must be taken not to overtax the liver with powerful cholagogues, instead using gentler herbs along with upregulating healthier organs of detoxification such as the kidneys. Likewise, if it's the kidneys that are diseased, more emphasis is placed upon the liver and bowels. Ideally, an herbal formula will contain all the categories of herbs used to support detoxification, including digestives, cholagogues, alteratives, aperients, diuretics and expectorants, in varying proportions depending on the requirements. An example formula is:

barberry root (cholagogue)	20 parts
cascara sagrada bark (aperient)	20 parts
red clover flower (alterative)	15 parts
dandelion leaf (diuretic)	15 parts
elecampane root (expectorant)	15 parts
ginger root (digestive)	15 parts
	100 parts

Dose

Tinctures: 5-10 mL (1-2 tsp) with water, 2-3x, daily before meals
Powders: 5-10 g (2-4 tsp) with water, 2-3x, daily before meals
Take for 10-14 days, along with a detoxification diet.

There are a number of proprietary detoxification formulas in the marketplace, and all of them follow this scheme to one degree or another, depending on the skill and knowledge of the formulator. Some are simple formulas whereas others are exceedingly complex. Look for products that have a basis in traditional herbal medicine, and are made from 100% organic or sustainably wildcrafted herbs.

In Ayurveda, one of the simplest formulas for detoxification is **triphala** powder, prepared from equal parts haritaki *(Terminalia chebula)*, bibhitaki *(Terminalia belerica)* and amalaki *(Phyllanthus emblica)*. According to Ayurveda triphala is both a rejuvenative (rasayana) and detoxifier (malashodhana), used on a regular basis to purify the body of wastes while boosting energy and balancing the nervous system. Triphala can be with an equal part licorice root *(Glycyrrhiza glabra)* if triphala alone is too drying, such as in vata conditions. Likewise, triphala can be mixed with equal parts aperient herbs such as cascara sagrada, turkey rhubarb or trivrit for a stronger, more laxative effect in constipation. Typical dose for triphala, whether mixed with other herbs or taken alone, is 3-5 grams, 2-3 times daily, mixed with water.

Section Five:
Therapeutic Diets

Therapeutic Diets

The following is a review of selected health conditions, each providing a basic overview of the doshas typically involved, dietary factors that provoke and inhibit the condition, and some key herbs already mentioned in this book that can be incorporated into the diet or taken as a supplement. It is not meant to be a complete review of each health issue nor represent all therapeutic options, but only provide some key elements when considering the role of food and herbs.

Food sensitivities and allergies

Various foods are well established to provoke a wide array of reactions in sensitive people, including everything from food sensitivities and food allergies, to full-blown pathologies such as celiac disease. Symptoms range from skin and digestive problems, to joint inflammation and neurological disorders. In this complex world, attempting to discern which foods provoke which reactions can be a difficult and tedious exercise, especially because some types of reactions occur several days or even weeks after consumption. To help the clinician sort through these factors, diagnostic tests such as the skin prick test, the radioallergosorbent test (RAST) and the enzyme-linked immunosorbent assay (ELISA) have been developed. While the skin-prick and radioallergosorbent tests are effective for isolating environmental allergies (e.g. pollen, animal dander, dust mites), they are less reliable when it comes to isolating potential food allergens. In recent years the ELISA has been developed as a way to test for food allergies, but its reliability and efficacy has come under question.[278] Other non-laboratory tests such as electroacupuncture ("vega-testing") and kinesiology ("muscle-testing") are sometimes used, but these have neither a scientific nor a historical, empirical basis.

The most effective method for determining if a particular food is playing a role in a health issue is to perform an **elimination-challenge diet**, completely eliminating the suspected food(s) from the diet for a period of 4-6 weeks. If and when the symptoms resolve, the food is re-introduced and any health changes are noted. I typically recommend the Paleolithic diet (p. 95) as a baseline diet to weed out the most common culprits, including casein (dairy), gluten (i.e. wheat, rye, barley, spelt, kamut) and soy.

List of health conditions

Acne
- pitta imbalance; autotoxicity (ama)
- pitta reducing diet (p. 100)
- check for food sensitivities, e.g. dairy, cereals (e.g. gluten), legumes (e.g. peanut, soy), eggs, citrus, beef, fish/shellfish, nuts and seeds, nightshades (e.g. potato, eggplant, tomato, bell pepper)
- avoid sugar, sweets, starchy foods, junk foods, and greasy foods
- implement a course of fasting and detoxification (p. 213)
- emphasize leafy greens, omega 3 fats (e.g. grass-fed meat/dairy, wild fish), fermented foods, vitamin D sources (e.g. oily fish, blood sausage, liver)
- useful herbs include amla, nettle, calendula, burdock root, dandelion root, turmeric, chickweed, peony and dang gui

Anemia
- vata imbalance
- vata reducing diet (p. 99)
- ensure good digestion; see **indigestion** (p. 241)
- caused by bleeding, autoimmunity, nutrient deficiencies, infection or toxins; can also be genetic (e.g. sickle cell anemia)
- if autoimmune, implement strict Paleolithic diet (p. 95)
- emphasize warming, nourishing soups and stews, iron-rich meats (e.g. goat, lamb, beef, poultry, eggs), stewed dried fruit (compote and syrups) and leafy greens cooked with fat
- useful herbs include amla, nettle, rehmannia, goji, dang gui, Szechuan pepper, tamarind, ashwagandha and Chinese red date

Arthritis

- vata imbalance; autotoxicity (ama); see **indigestion** (p. 241)
- vata reducing diet (p. 99)
- implement a course of fasting and detoxification (p. 213)
- eliminate sticky, heavy and hard to digest foods including flour products, sweets, dairy and deep-fried foods
- check for food sensitivities, e.g. dairy, cereals (e.g. gluten), legumes (e.g. peanut, soy), eggs, citrus, beef, fish/shellfish, nuts and seeds, nightshades (e.g. potato, eggplant, tomato, capsicum)
- emphasize anti-inflammatory foods including oily fish, grass-fed meat/dairy, leafy greens and vegetables
- ensure mineral-rich foods, including bone/seaweed broth, mineral water
- ensure adequate vitamin D3 consumption, e.g. oily fish, blood sausage
- avoid alcohol, coffee and tea
- useful herbs include turmeric, ginger, juniper, ashwagandha, pippali, garlic, cumin, caraway, dandelion root, fenugreek, ajwain and nettle

Asthma

- vata-kapha imbalance; autotoxicity (ama); see **food allergies** (p. 237), **indigestion** (p. 241)
- vata and kapha reducing diets (pp. 99/101)
- avoid kapha-promoting foods, e.g. sugar, sweets, dairy, flour products, refined oils, deep-fried food
- check for food sensitivities, e.g. dairy, cereals (e.g. gluten), legumes (e.g. peanut, soy), eggs, citrus, beef, fish/shellfish, nuts and seeds, nightshades (e.g. potato, eggplant, tomato, capsicum)
- implement a course of fasting and detoxification (p. 213)
- emphasize leafy-greens, oily fish, grass-fed meat/dairy, spicy-warming foods, and half-sweet antioxidant-rich fruits
- useful herbs and spices include thyme, hing, holy basil, rosemary, garlic, cayenne, oregano, cinnamon, turmeric, amla and ginger

Colds and cough

- kapha imbalance; autotoxicity (ama); see **indigestion** (p. 241)
- kapha reducing diet (p. 101)
- dry cough indicates vata; yellow-green mucus or blood indicates pitta
- avoid kapha-promoting foods, e.g. sugar, sweets, dairy, flour products, refined oils, deep-fried food
- implement a course of fasting and detoxification (p. 213)
- rehydrate the body with non-fatty soups and stews (e.g. broth, kitchari), steamed vegetables
- useful herbs and spices include ginger, holy basil, garlic, cayenne, thyme and oregano, taken with honey
- for dry cough include herbs such as pear skin, Solomon's seal, peony root, lily bulb and Chinese yam
- for pitta (heat) symptoms include herbs such as amla, calendula, chickweed and nettle

Constipation

- vata imbalance; autotoxicity (ama); see **indigestion** (p. 241)
- vata reducing diet (p. 99)
- eliminate sticky and heavy foods that impair gut motility, including flour products, sweets, dairy and deep-fried foods
- implement a course of fasting and detoxification (p. 213)
- emphasize live-culture fermented foods to restore gut ecology
- rehydrate the digestive system with fatty soups and stews
- emphasize high fiber foods such as whole grains, leafy greens, root, vegetables, stewed fruit and hemp seed
- useful herbs include turmeric, fenugreek, amla, astragalus, codonopsis, orange peel, garlic, caraway, fennel and ginger
- for constipation caused by dryness, useful herbs include shatavari, Solomon's seal, lily bulb, peony root, Chinese yam, slippery elm or hemp seed

Dementia

- vata imbalance; see **heart disease** (p. 239)
- vata reducing diet (p. 99)

- eliminate refined carbohydrates, sweets and sugar, deep-fried foods
- avoid MSG, artificial sweeteners, food additives
- emphasize nourishing, easily digestible foods including soups and stews
- include fermented foods to promote good digestion
- ensure optimal protein and fat intake, omega 3 fats
- emphasize antioxidant-rich fruits and vegetables, e.g. blueberry, leafy greens, beets, purple cabbage, yellow squash, etc.
- useful herbs include rosemary, ashwagandha, amla, turmeric, ginger, ginseng, holy basil, cayenne and gotu kola

Depression
- vata imbalance; see **indigestion** (p. 241), **food allergies** (p. 237, **anemia** (p. 232)
- vata reducing diet (p. 99)
- eliminate refined carbohydrates, sweets and sugar
- check for food sensitivities, e.g. dairy, cereals (e.g. gluten), legumes (e.g. peanut, soy), eggs, citrus, beef, fish/shellfish, nuts and seeds, nightshades (e.g. potato, eggplant, tomato, capsicum)
- implement a course of fasting and detoxification (p. 213)
- avoid alcohol
- emphasize grounding, nourishing foods that are easily digestible, e.g. soups and stews, steamed vegetables
- ensure vitamin D sources, e.g. oily fish, pork fat, blood sausage
- ensure adequate protein and omega 3 fats
- useful herbs include ashwagandha, goji, American ginseng, amla, holy basil, rose, fennel, juniper, lily bulb, rosemary and gotu kola

Diabetes (adult onset)
- vata-kapha imbalance; see **indigestion** (p. 241), **obesity** (p. 243), **heart disease** (p. 239)
- avoid all sweets, sugars and starchy foods
- implement a strict low-carbohydrate, Paleolithic diet (p. 95), emphasizing high quality fats and proteins, and an

equal or greater volume of non-starchy vegetables at each meal
- limit fruit to a single small serving of half-sweet, antioxidant-rich fruits such as blueberry, guava, passionfruit, raspberry, etc.
- useful herbs include fenugreek, amla, cinnamon, ginseng, garlic, turmeric, holy basil, pippali, bitter melon, astragalus and ashwagandha

Diarrhea
- pitta imbalance; autotoxicity (ama)
- pitta reducing diet (p. 100)
- avoid spicy and greasy foods
- for chronic conditions check for food sensitivities, e.g. dairy, cereals (e.g. gluten), legumes (e.g. peanut, soy), eggs, citrus, beef, fish/shellfish, nuts and seeds, nightshades (e.g. potato, eggplant, tomato, bell pepper)
- restore electrolytes with salted broth, soup and rice dishes (e.g. kitchari, congee)
- as symptoms improve add fermented foods to restore gut ecology
- useful herbs include dill, fennel, ginger, caraway, cardamom, hing, turmeric, cinnamon, carob, coriander, nettle and pink salt

Eczema
- pitta-kapha imbalance; autotoxicity (ama); see **indigestion** (p. 241)
- kapha and pitta reducing diets (pp. 100/101)
- avoid spicy and very dry or greasy foods
- eliminate refined carbohydrates, sweets and sugar
- check for food sensitivities, e.g. dairy, cereals (e.g. gluten), legumes (e.g. peanut, soy), eggs, citrus, beef, fish/shellfish, nuts and seeds, nightshades (e.g. potato, eggplant, tomato, capsicum)
- implement a course of fasting and detoxification (p. 213)
- emphasize omega 3 fats (oily fish, grass-fed meat/dairy), leafy greens and vegetables
- useful herbs include burdock, nettle, turmeric, gotu kola, lemonbalm, prickly ash, ginger, pippali, calendula, chickweed and juniper

Fever
- pitta imbalance; autotoxicity (ama)
- pitta reducing diet (p. 100)
- avoid solid foods
- ensure adequate hydration with non-fat lightly salted broth
- useful herbs include ginger, turmeric, cayenne, lemonbalm, Szechuan pepper, coriander, oregano, basil and thyme
- after the fever has resolved, follow the measures listed under **indigestion**

Fibromyalgia
- vata imbalance; autotoxicity (ama); see **indigestion** (p. 241), **arthritis** (p. 233)
- linked to autoimmune disease; implement strict Paleolithic diet (p. 95)
- implement a course of fasting and detoxification (p. 213)
- emphasize omega 3 fats (oily fish, grass-fed animal produce) and leafy greens
- useful herbs include ashwagandha, American ginseng, nutmeg, turmeric, ginger and amla

Food allergies
- kapha imbalance; autotoxicity (ama); see **indigestion** (p. 241)
- kapha reducing diet (p. 101)
- implement a course of fasting and detoxification (p. 213)
- check for food sensitivities, e.g. dairy, cereals (e.g. gluten), legumes (e.g. peanut, soy), eggs, citrus, beef, fish/shellfish, nuts and seeds, nightshades (e.g. potato, eggplant, tomato, capsicum)
- avoid kapha-promoting foods, e.g. flour products, dairy, sugar, sweets, yeasted foods, wine, beer
- avoid packaged foods, junk foods, food additives and preservatives
- emphasize easily digestible foods such as soups, stews, steamed vegetables, fermented foods
- useful herbs include ginger, turmeric, hing, holy basil, cardamom, cumin, caraway, dill, coriander, fenugreek, mint, pippali and nettle

Gallstones

- vata-pitta imbalance; see **obesity** (p. 244), **indigestion** (p. 241)
- vata and pitta reducing diets (p. 99)
- follow the rules of food-combining (p. 29)
- check for food sensitivities, e.g. dairy, cereals (e.g. gluten), legumes (e.g. peanut, soy), eggs, citrus, beef, fish/shellfish, nuts and seeds, nightshades (e.g. potato, eggplant, tomato, capsicum)
- eliminate flour products and refined oils from the diet
- ensure adequate fiber consumption, emphasizing whole grains and vegetables
- ensure proper hydration, emphasizing soups, stews, steamed vegetables and herbal teas (nettle, dandelion, cleavers)
- useful herbs include turmeric, mint, orange peel, coriander, caraway, amla, shatavari and bitter melon

Gout

- vata-pitta imbalance; autotoxicity (ama); see **arthritis** (p. 233)
- vata and pitta reducing diets (p. 99)
- follow the rules of food-combining (p. 29)
- avoid alcohol and sugar, which blocks purine excretion
- implement a course of fasting and detoxification (p. 213)
- linked to autoimmune disease; implement strict Paleolithic diet (p. 95)
- limit purine-rich foods including animal proteins, legumes and shellfish
- emphasize vegetables and leafy greens to alkalize the blood
- useful herbs include turmeric, ginger, amla, triphala, ashwagandha, dandelion, burdock, nettle and chickweed

Hay fever

- vata-kapha imbalance; autotoxicity (ama); see **food allergies** (p. 237)
- vata and kapha reducing diets (pp. 99/101)
- usually concurrent with wheat and dairy sensitivities
- implement a course of fasting and detoxification (p. 213), prior to hay fever season

- avoid congesting, ama-producing foods, e.g. flour products, dairy, sugar, sweets, yeasted foods, greasy meat and deep-fried foods
- increase consumption of leafy greens and antioxidant-rich fruits
- ensure adequate hydration with teas, soups and stews
- useful herbs include pippali, amla, turmeric, ginger, holy basil, bay leaf, cardamom, codonopsis, astragalus, orange peel, garlic, nettle, mint, sage and cayenne

Heart disease (arterial disease, high cholesterol)
- vata imbalance; see **diabetes** (p. 235) and **obesity** (p. 243)
- vata reducing diet (p. 99)
- reduce sugar, sweets and starchy foods
- avoid refined oils, deep-fried food, grain-fed (feed-lot) meat
- avoid excessive alcohol, coffee and tea
- emphasize grass-fed and wild animal products
- emphasize leafy-greens and half-sweet antioxidant-rich fruits
- ensure vitamin D sources, e.g. oily fish, pork fat, blood sausage
- useful herbs include rosemary, garlic, cayenne, oregano, astragalus, amla, cinnamon, turmeric, fenugreek, holy basil and ginger

Heartburn and hiatus hernia
- vata-pitta imbalance
- vata and pitta reducing diets (p. 99)
- relates to impaired gut motility; see **indigestion** (p. 241), **constipation** (p. 234), **obesity** (p. 243)
- follow the rules of food-combining (p. 29)
- avoid sticky, heavy and hard to digest foods including flour products, dairy, sweets and greasy foods
- avoid very spicy herbs that can aggravate reflux, e.g. cayenne, ginger, peppermint, garlic, onion, horseradish
- avoid alcohol
- emphasize high fiber foods including vegetables and whole grains
- useful herbs to soothe esophageal inflammation include slippery elm, licorice, chickweed and calendula

- useful herbs to promote motility include turmeric, dandelion root, triphala and coriander

Hemorrhoids
- vata imbalance; often with pitta or kapha component
- relates to **indigestion** (p. 241), **constipation** (vata, p. 234) or **diarrhea** (pitta, p. 236), **food allergies** (kapha, p. 237)
- avoid sticky, heavy and hard to digest foods including flour products, dairy, sweets and greasy foods
- ensure adequate consumption of high fiber foods including leafy greens and whole grains
- useful foods include black sesame seed and buttermilk (khadi) (p. 177)
- emphasize antioxidant-rich fruits such as blueberry, bilberry, raspberry, amla, hawthorn and cranberry
- emphasize fermented foods to promote a healthy gut ecology
- useful herbs include turmeric, dandelion root, burdock root, triphala and fenugreek

Hyperactivity
- vata imbalance
- vata reducing diet (p. 99)
- avoid sugar, sweets, starchy foods
- check for food sensitivities, e.g. dairy, cereals (e.g. gluten), legumes (e.g. peanut, soy), eggs, citrus, beef, fish/shellfish, nuts and seeds, nightshades (e.g. potato, eggplant, tomato, capsicum)
- avoid MSG, artificial sweeteners, food additives
- emphasize nourishing grounding foods (animal proteins and fats), fermented foods, leafy greens and whole grains
- useful herbs include ashwagandha, gotu kola, rehmannia, amla, lemonbalm, Chinese red dates, goji, lily bulb, poria and shiitake mushroom

Hypoglycemia
- vata imbalance
- vata reducing diet (p. 99)
- follow the rules of food quantity and timing (p. 28); ensure a good breakfast

- avoid all refined flour products, sweets, sugar and sweet fruits
- avoid alcohol, coffee and tea
- check for food sensitivities, e.g. dairy, cereals (e.g. gluten), legumes (e.g. peanut, soy), eggs, citrus, beef, fish/shellfish, nuts and seeds, nightshades (e.g. potato, eggplant, tomato, capsicum)
- emphasize high fat, high protein meals, with fiber-rich foods, e.g. leafy greens, root vegetables, whole grains
- ensure mineral-rich foods, including bone/seaweed broth, mineral water
- useful herbs include ashwagandha, ginger, American ginseng, goji, turmeric, rehmannia, dang gui, licorice and peony

Hypothyroidism
- vata-kapha imbalance; see **obesity** (p. 244), **indigestion** (p. 241)
- vata and kapha-reducing diets (pp. 99/101)
- may relate to excessive consumption of goitrogens (i.e. turnips, cabbage, mustard, cassava root, soy, peanuts, pine nuts and millet)
- linked to autoimmune disease; implement strict Paleolithic diet (p. 95)
- ensure adequate mineral intake including iodine, e.g. seaweed, bone broths, mineral water, herbs and spices
- useful herbs include cayenne, ginger, codonopsis, astragalus, pippali, orange peel, cinnamon, cardamom, Szechuan pepper, American ginseng, fenugreek, ginseng and ashwagandha

Indigestion
- kapha imbalance
- kapha reducing diet (p. 101)
- ensure diet is appropriate to the current season (p. 26)
- follow the rules of food quantity and timing (p. 28)
- follow the rules of food-combining (p. 29)
- avoid sticky, heavy and hard to digest foods including flour products, dairy, sweets and greasy foods
- ensure consumption of live-culture fermented foods (p. 124)

- useful herbs include ginger, fennel, turmeric, astragalus, codonopsis, fenugreek, orange peel, pippali, cardamom and cayenne

Infertility
- vata imbalance; autotoxicity (ama)
- vata reducing diet (p. 99)
- implement a course of fasting and detoxification (p. 213)
- check for food sensitivities, e.g. dairy, cereals (e.g. gluten), legumes (e.g. peanut, soy), eggs, citrus, beef, fish/shellfish, nuts and seeds, nightshades (e.g. potato, eggplant, tomato, capsicum)
- eliminate all packaged and refined foods
- avoid alcohol, coffee and tea
- emphasize nourishing fertility-enhancing foods such as wild or grass-fed animal meat, dairy and fish, prepared with medicinal herbs as soups and stews; leafy greens and root vegetables
- useful herbs include ashwagandha, American ginseng, shatavari, ginseng, dang gui, peony, Chinese yam, poria, licorice, amla, nettle, cinnamon, nutmeg, ginger, sesame seed and goji

Inflammatory bowel disease
- vata-pitta imbalance; see **indigestion** (p. 241), **diarrhea** (p. 236) and **food allergies** (p. 237)
- autoimmune disease; implement strict Paleolithic diet (p. 95)
- avoid alcohol, coffee and tea
- restore electrolytes with salted broth and soup, slowly building up complexity in the diet
- follow the rules of food-combining (p. 29)
- as symptoms improve add in fermented foods to restore gut ecology
- useful herbs include slippery elm, licorice, astragalus, codonopsis, coriander, American ginseng, shatavari, calendula, fenugreek, turmeric, ginger and nettle

Insomnia
- vata-pitta imbalance; see **indigestion** (p. 241)
- vata and pitta reducing diets (p. 99)

- avoid sweets and sugars that promote large alterations in blood sugar
- avoid stimulants, e.g. coffee, tea, chocolate, chili
- emphasize high fat/protein meals, especially for breakfast
- boiled milk before bed
- useful herbs include ashwagandha, nutmeg, poria, gotu kola and poppy seed

Kidney stones (calcium oxalate stones)
- vata-kapha imbalance
- vata and kapha reducing diets (pp. 99/101)
- ensure adequate hydration, e.g. water, soups, steamed vegetables, coconut water
- enhance consumption of fiber-rich foods including leafy greens and non-starchy vegetables, root vegetables and whole grains
- reduce salt, meat, milk and protein consumption
- eliminate sugar, alcohol, tea, coffee and dairy consumption
- reduce oxalate-containing foods (e.g. rhubarb, spinach)
- increase magnesium-containing foods (e.g. barley, sesame, coconut, avocado)
- useful foods include red adzuki bean and chicken gizzard
- useful herbs include dandelion leaf, poria, calendula, juniper, nettle, chickweed, parsley and ajwain

Menopause
- vata-pitta imbalance
- vata and pitta reducing diets (p. 99)
- avoid spicy, heating foods, e.g. chili, garlic, ginger, citrus
- emphasize moistening, nourishing foods, e.g. soups, stews, steamed vegetables
- emphasize leafy greens, sprouts and legumes as supplemental phytoestrogen sources
- useful herbs include American ginseng, dang gui, shatavari, goji, astragalus, chickweed, nettle, dandelion, Chinese yam, lily bulb, sage, peony and rehmannia

Obesity
- kapha imbalance; see **indigestion** (p. 241), **diabetes** (p. 235) and **heart disease** (p. 239)

- kapha reducing diet (p. 101)
- avoid refined sweets, starches, flour products, deep-fried foods
- emphasize light, easily digestible foods, lean proteins, omega 3 fats (e.g. wild fish, grass-fed meat/dairy), fermented foods
- emphasize calorie-dense foods with an equal volume of non-starchy vegetables
- increase consumption of fiber-rich foods, e.g. wild rice, quinoa, legumes
- useful herbs include basil, bay, black mustard, black pepper, pippali, cardamom, cayenne, fenugreek, cumin, ginger, garlic, holy basil, juniper, turmeric and poria

Osteoporosis
- vata imbalance; see **arthritis** (p. 233)
- vata reducing diet (p. 99)
- emphasize nourishing foods such as bone and seaweed broths, leafy greens, high quality fats and proteins, stewed fruits, fermented foods
- ensure vitamin D sources, e.g. oily fish, pork fat, blood sausage
- useful herbs include ashwagandha, ginseng, shatavari, seaweed, he shou wu, garlic, dang gui, peony, goji, Chinese red dates, astragalus and amla

Parasites
- kapha imbalance; autotoxicity (ama)
- kapha reducing diet (p. 101)
- implement a course of fasting and detoxification (p. 213)
- avoid sugar, sweets, starchy and greasy foods
- emphasize light, easily digestible foods such as soups, grain and legume dishes and steamed vegetables
- use fermented foods after treatment to restore gut ecology
- useful herbs include garlic, cayenne, hing, dill, epazote, ginger, mustard, clove, turmeric and ajwain

Post-partum exhaustion
- vata imbalance; see **anemia** (p. 232), **depression** (p. 235)
- vata reducing diet (p. 99)

- emphasize nourishing soups and stews, iron-rich meats (e.g. goat, lamb, beef, poultry, eggs), stewed dried fruit (compote and syrups), fortified wines, and leafy greens cooked with fat
- useful herbs include American ginseng, amla, nettle, rehmannia, goji, dang gui, ashwagandha, Chinese red date, astragalus, shatavari, cinnamon, goji, Solomon's seal and peony

Premenstrual Syndrome
- vata imbalance; relates to **indigestion** (p. 241)
- vata reducing diet (p. 99)
- check for food sensitivities, e.g. dairy, cereals (e.g. gluten), legumes (e.g. peanut, soy), eggs, citrus, beef, fish/shellfish, nuts and seeds, nightshades (e.g. potato, eggplant, tomato, capsicum)
- eliminate refined oils
- ensure omega 3 fat consumption (e.g. grass-fed meat/dairy and poultry, oily wild fish)
- replace sugar and sweets with high fat, high protein foods; see **hypoglycemia**
- ensure proper bowel ecology by increasing fiber intake, e.g. leafy greens, root vegetables, whole grains; fermented foods
- useful herbs include nettle, dandelion root, American ginseng, rehmannia, goji, dang gui, shatavari, ashwagandha, turmeric, ginger, peony, amla, rose and he shou wu

Prostatitis
- vata-kapha imbalance; see **indigestion** (p. 241)
- vata and kapha reducing diets (pp. 99/101)
- check for food sensitivities, e.g. gluten, soy, dairy, legumes, nuts, cereals, eggs
- eliminate alcohol, coffee and tea
- ensure proper bowel ecology by increasing fiber intake, e.g. leafy greens, root vegetables, whole grains; fermented foods
- ensure adequate consumption of omega 3 fats (e.g. wild and grass-fed meat, dairy and fish)

- useful herbs include dandelion leaf, chickweed, nettle, ashwagandha, juniper, parsley, ginseng, rehmannia and poria

Ulcers

- vata-pitta imbalance; see **heartburn** (p. 239), **indigestion** (p. 241)
- vata and pitta reducing diets (p. 99)
- check for food sensitivities, e.g. dairy, cereals (e.g. gluten), legumes (e.g. peanut, soy), eggs, citrus, beef, fish/shellfish, nuts and seeds, nightshades (e.g. potato, eggplant, tomato, capsicum)
- follow the rules of food-combining (p. 29)
- eliminate alcohol, coffee and tea
- avoid very spicy herbs, e.g. cayenne, ginger, peppermint, garlic
- emphasize fiber-rich foods including vegetables such as cabbage, chard, kale and beets
- fermented foods can be added later in the healing process
- useful herbs to soothe inflammation and promote healing include slippery elm, licorice, chickweed, calendula, turmeric, dandelion root and amla

Conclusion

A few last words...

To understand the theory and practice of food, like that of medicine, takes time, effort and skill. None of us are born with an instruction manual and so we all start from the beginning. And the beginning place is the hardest. Imagine the effort and perseverance required by the first plants of spring, like the alpine Pasqueflower (*Anenome pulsatilla*) that must rise up and break through ice and snow to meet with the sun. An ancient Chinese text called the *Yi Jing* states that the beginning of any endeavor is a time of confusion and questions, of running hither and thither, but if we exert some perseverance we can create order from chaos. The *Yi Jing* tells us that it may take some time, and it may require some help, but it can be done.

To properly understand food you must have an interest in the support of life, whether it's your life, your family's life, your community, or the health of the planet. There needs to be a reason to connect with something beyond the narrow limitations of your being. Although we find fulfillment in relationships, art and science, perhaps all we are looking for is a connection to life. And there is no deeper connection to life than food. Unlike the science of modern nutrition, the theory and practice of food begins with the senses – but to begin this journey they must be awoken. We must overthrow the yoke of bland industrial mediocrity thrust upon us as nourishment, and take back our birthright, which is to be nourished by this earth in all its diversity. We have a right to choose quality over quantity. It is our right to eat, and protecting it is the most fundamental of acts. Not to hoard but to share, because food is sharing. Eating is sharing. Food is life! Let the myriad beings share in the delight and nourishment of eating!

In this book I have tried to provide a model of food and eating, but like all models it has its limitations. It is meant to be a representation of life, a tool you can use to restore balance, but it is not life itself. For that you need to look at yourself. Let go of the thinking mind and listen to your body and the inherent wisdom it contains. If your experiences support the information in this book, then I have achieved my goal. I profess no ultimate truth except your quiet confidence – peaceful and self-resplendent – the knowledge that you, dear reader, already contain the wisdom you seek. The knowledge is already there: listen to the food, listen to your body.

Beyond the issue of nourishment the most frequent issue I see in my clinic is loneliness. People living alone or otherwise separate lives. Weighed down with a myriad number of responsibilities they never have time to nourish themselves. Instead they seek fast food alternatives or gimmicky appliances that are supposed to be quick and easy when they are really just cheap and plastic. At one time the kitchen was the heart of the home but now for many it is an empty and meticulously "germ-free" epitaph to nourishment, more like a mini-warehouse of industrial foods than a place where life gets made. Since the very beginning of time there was at the center of every home at least one person who kept the fires burning. For me, it was my French Canadian grandfather Philogene. Although he died when I was five years old, I clearly remember his big vegetable garden and the abundant fruit trees and bushes in his yard. I remember standing bare feet in the soil, eating a fresh carrot he pulled from the garden. I remember him siphoning and decanting homemade wine, baking bread, making tourtière (meat pie), collecting sand for the garden on the banks of the Fraser river, and tending to his much-admired roses. I remember lots of activity in the kitchen, family and friends dropping by for a visit, sometimes in the evenings to collect around the piano, to sing songs and drink a little homemade wine. Some of you may have similar memories, and if you are lucky you are carrying on this tradition. But many of you have no memory of anything like this, or if you do, they are only memories and nothing more. The home-fire has been put out. The symbol of home, good health and vitality is gone.

Although it has traditionally been the woman's role to keep the home fire burning, as my grandfather proved, gender is not important. But in modern times, when everyone works or goes to school, the subject of nourishment can no longer be only one person's responsibility. If the internet has taught us anything, it is that we are all part of a vast network. Life is a network, food is a network. This is the thing we need to understand. There is no real separation between us and food, and thus food is everyone's responsibility. Let us join together in the kitchen, where nourishment becomes everyone's responsibility. Man, woman, husband, wife, boy, girl, sister, brother – friends and new families – all come together and partake. Let's leverage our potential and make the practice of food easy and quick, not because it doesn't take time, but because when we work together we are so much more efficient. Refuse to live a lonely isolated life of partial self-nourishment. Come together in the celebration of life and bring the food and the people back into the home. Let's open our kitchens to each other, and like a plant sink our roots deep into the earth to realize that we all arise from this same dark soil. Eating food, becoming food. We are all part of this cycle. We are nourishment. We are food.

Appendices

Appendix I: Constitution

This is a chart you can use to determine your physical constitution (prakriti), discussed on page 16. Total up your scores to see which dosha(s) dominate, dividing each score by 21 to calculate the percentages.

Physical features	Vata	Pitta	Kapha
Describe your frame size.	Small bones; thin; little fat, or localized to abdomen only; bones, tendons and veins otherwise prominent ☐	Average bones, neither thin nor heavy; little fat, or localized to abdomen only; muscular ☐	Large-boned; heavy; bones, tendons and veins covered in a layer of fat ☐
How much did you weigh in your early 20's?	Low Women: < 105 lbs Men: < 130 lbs ☐	Average Women: 105-135 lbs Men: 140-180 lbs ☐	Heavy Women: > 135 lbs Men: > 180 lbs ☐
Describe your complexion.	Dull, pale, greyish ☐	Red, ruddy or flushed ☐	Pink, pale, whitish ☐
Describe the quality of your skin and mucus membranes.	Dry, thin, cold, rough, cracked ☐	Warm, moist, pink-red, flushed, hot ☐	Thick, pale, greasy, cold, soft, smooth ☐
Describe the quality of your hair.	Coarse, kinky, unruly, dry ☐	Fine, thin, soft, moist ☐	Heavy, thick, oily ☐
Describe your head.	Small ☐	Average ☐	Large ☐
Describe your forehead.	Small ☐	High ☐	Average ☐
Describe your eyebrows.	Small, thin ☐	Average, fine ☐	Thick, bushy ☐
Describe your eyelashes.	Small, short ☐	Average, fine ☐	Thick, long ☐
Describe your eyes.	Small, dry, grey ☐	Average, piercing, bright, reddish ☐	Large, moist, white ☐
Describe your nose.	Small, uneven, thin septum ☐	Average, angular shape, medium septum ☐	Large, thick, wide septum ☐
Describe your lips.	Thin, small, dry, bluish ☐	Average, red ☐	Large, thick, pale ☐
Describe your teeth and gums.	Thin, uneven, gums pale ☐	Teeth average; gums red ☐	Teeth large and thick, gums pink ☐
Describe your shoulders and arms.	Thin, small ☐	Average ☐	Large, thick, broad ☐
Describe your chest.	Thin, small, narrow ☐	Average, muscular ☐	Thick, large, broad ☐
Describe your hips/pelvis.	Thin, small, narrow ☐	Average ☐	Large, broad, thick ☐

Describe your hands.	Thin, rough, ☐	Muscular, average ☐	Large, thick ☐
Describe your nails.	Thin, breaks easily, fissured ☐	Soft, quickly growing ☐	Thick, hard, smooth ☐
Describe your legs.	Thin, small ☐	Average, muscular ☐	Large, thick ☐
Describe your feet.	Thin, small ☐	Average, muscular ☐	Large, thick ☐
Describe your body hair.	Sparse, coarse, dry ☐	Thin, fine, moist ☐	Thick, moist ☐
TOTAL	9 /21 points	9 /21 points	3 /21 points
Percentage of each dosha (divide by 21)	%	%	%

Appendix II: Meal Plans

The following are meal plans for the Paleolithic diet (page 95), and both the vegetarian and non-vegetarian Ayurveda diets (page 98). These meal plans draw upon many of the recipes found in this book (in bold), and are meant to create a model that will inspire you to create your own approach. In the real world you will likely have leftovers, and if eaten within a day or so after preparation, ensuring proper storage, can be incorporated into future meals, such as lunch the next day. For single people especially I have them make use of slow-cookers and pressure cookers, making big batches of food that they can portion off and then store in the freezer until needed. This is also a good approach for busy families.

To determine portion size, please review the section on Food Quantity and Timing, page 28. Remember that any meal plan is best punctuated by periodic fasting (p. 219) to restore and balance the metabolism.

Paleolithic Diet Meal Plan

Meal	Day One	Day Two	Day Three	Day Four	Day Five
Breakfast (8-9 am)	Basted eggs, sautéed onion, zucchini and sundried tomato, steamed buttercup squash	**Poached Herb Wild Salmon**, steamed assorted vegetables	Grilled steak and eggs with **Garlic-Basil Rapini**	Scrambled eggs with **Salsa**, sliced avocado, steamed chard	Baked lamb sausages, **Old-fashioned Sauerkraut**, steamed broccoli with **Garlic Herb Oil**
Snack (2-3 pm)	Fruit	Bison jerky	Fruit	Salmon jerky	Pickled mackerel
Supper (5-7 pm)	**Persian Lamb Shanks** with grilled zucchini, eggplant, pepper, onion and parsnips	Mediterranean-Rub roasted chicken, roasted vegetables and garlic, steamed chard	**Five-Spice Bison Stew**, baked butternut squash, **Chinese Greens and Arame**	**Goat Curry**, **Spicy Saag**, **Carrot Pickle**	Salmon and tuna sashimi, kale-wakame salad, **Gomashio**

Ayurveda Diet: Non-vegetarian Meal Plan

Meal	Day One	Day Two	Day Three	Day Four	Day Five
Breakfast (8-9am)	Muttar panir, Roti, stir-fried leafy greens	Vegetable omelet, sliced avocado, Salsa	Breakfast Bowl	Scrambled eggs with Salsa, sliced avocado, steamed chard	Kitchari, Carrot Pickle, Coconut Chutney
Lunch (12-2 pm)	Garden Vegetable Soup, Greek salad	Borscht, sour cream	Mulligatawny Soup, Roti	Garden Vegetable soup, salad	Rosemary Oat Cakes, Pickled Pepper Paste goat cheese, cucumber
Snack (3-4pm)	Smoked mackerel	Tamari seeds	Fruit	Tamari seeds	Fruit
Supper (5-7 pm)	Persian Lamb Shanks, steamed chard, Brown Basmati Pullao	Poached Herb Wild Salmon, steamed assorted vegetables, Northwest Wild Rice	Mexican Chicken Stew, corn tortillas (w/lime), Salsa, steamed kale	Mediterranean Rub roast chicken, Garlic Basil Rapini, roasted baby potatoes with rosemary	Five-Spice Bison Stew, Chinese Greens and Arame, Goji Quinoa Pilaf

Ayurveda Diet: Vegetarian Meal Plan

Meal	Day One	Day Two	Day Three	Day Four	Day Five
Breakfast (8-9 am)	Urad-mung Dhal, methi Thepla, Yoghurt raita	Vegetable omelet, sliced avocado, Salsa	Kitchari, sautéed vegetables, Indian Carrot Pickle	Brown Basmati Pullao, chickpea dhal, steamed greens with ghee	Breakfast Bowl
Lunch (12-2 pm)	Borscht, sour cream	Rosemary Oat Cakes, goat feta, sliced cucumber, Pickled Pepper Paste	Garden Vegetable Soup, Old-fashioned Sauerkraut	Garden Vegetable Soup, Roti	Scrambled eggs, stir-fried onion, zucchini and cilantro, goat feta
Snack (3-4pm)	Oat Cakes with Cultured Butter	Fruit	Mango Chat	Fruit	Tamari Seeds
Supper	Asian kitchari, Ginger-Tamari Squash, brown rice, Kimchi	Gobi Parantha, Coconut Chutney	Khadi, Brown Basmati Pullao, Spicy Saag	Greek Salad, roasted sweet potatoes with Garlic Herb Oil	Muttar panir, Roti

Appendix III: Vegetables

Vegetables are cold, light and wet in quality, and in general, help to reduce pitta (inflammation) and congestion (kapha). When cooked and mixed with some kind of fat or oil (e.g. butter, olive oil) most vegetables also reduce vata. Vegetables that are hot in nature tend to enhance digestion and increase pitta. For more information please refer to page 38.

The effect on vata (V), pitta (P) and kapha (K) is noted as an increasing (+), decreasing (-) or neutral (=) effect.

Vegetables	Flavor	Quality	Doshas
Amaranth greens	bitter	cold, light, dry	KP-, V+
Artichoke	bitter, sweet	cold, light, wet	KP-, V+
Arugula	bitter	cold, light, wet	KP-, V+
Asparagus	sweet, bitter	cold, heavy, wet	VP-, K+
Avocado	sweet	cold, heavy, wet	VP-, K+
Bamboo shoot	sweet, bitter	cold, heavy, wet	VP-, K+
Beet greens	bitter	cold, light, wet	KP-, V+
Beet root	sweet, bitter	cold, heavy, wet	VPK=
Bell pepper	sweet, pungent	hot, light, wet	VK-, P=
Bitter gourd (karela, ku gua)	bitter	cold, light, dry	PK-, V+
Bok choy	bitter	cold, light, dry	KP-, V+
Broccoli	bitter	cold, light, dry	KP-, V+
Brussels sprout	bitter	cold, light, dry	KP-, V+
Burdock root (gobo)	bitter, sweet	cold, light, dry	KP-, V+
Cabbage	bitter, pungent	cold, light, dry	KP-, V+
Carrot	sweet, bitter	hot, light, wet	VK-, P=
Cassava	sweet, bitter	hot, heavy, wet	VPK+
Cauliflower	bitter	cold, light, dry	KP-, V+
Celery	salty	cold, heavy, wet	VPK=
Chard	bitter	cold, light, dry	KP-, V+
Chickweed	bitter	cold, light, dry	KP-, V+
Chives	pungent	hot, light, wet	K-, VP+
Collard greens	bitter	cold, light, dry	KP-, V+
Corn (sweet)	sweet	cold, heavy, dry	P-, VK+
Cucumber	sweet, bitter	cold, heavy, wet	VP-, K+
Daikon	pungent	hot, light, dry	K-, VP+
Dandelion	bitter	cold, light, dry	KP-, V+
Eggplant	sweet, pungent	hot, light, dry	VK-, P+
Endive	bitter	cold, light, dry	KP-, V+
Gai lan	bitter	cold, light, dry	KP-, V+
Garlic	pungent, sweet	hot, heavy, wet	VK-, P+

Ginger	pungent	hot, light, dry	VK-, P+
Kale	bitter	cold, light, dry	KP-, V+
Kohlrabi	sweet, bitter	cold, light, dry	KP-, V+
Lambsquarters	bitter	cold, light, dry	PK-, V+
Leek	pungent, sweet	hot, light, wet	VK-, P+
Lettuce	bitter	cold, light, dry	KP-, V+
Lotus root	sweet, astringent	cold, light, dry	P-, VK+
Mushroom	sweet	cold, heavy, wet	PV-, K+
Mustard	pungent, bitter	hot, light, dry	K-, VP+
Nettle	bitter, astringent	cold, light, dry	PK-, V+
Onion	pungent, sweet	hot, heavy, wet	VK-, P+
Pak choy	bitter	cold, light, dry	PK-, V+
Parsnip	sweet, bitter	hot, heavy, dry	K-, VP+
Pea sprouts	bitter	cold, light, dry	PK-, V+
Potato	sweet, astringent	hot, heavy, dry	V-, PK+
Pumpkin	sweet	hot, heavy, wet	V-, PK+
Purslane	sour	hot, light, dry	PK-, V+
Radicchio	bitter	cold, light, dry	PK-, V+
Radish	pungent, sweet	hot, light, dry	K-, VP+
Rutabaga, turnip	sweet, pungent, bitter	cold, light, dry	PK-, V+
Sea vegetables	salty	hot, heavy, wet	VK-, P+
Shallot	pungent, sweet	hot, light, wet	VK-, P+
Sorrel	sour	hot, light, dry	VK-, P+
Spinach	sour, bitter	cold, light, dry	P-, VK+
Sui choy	bitter, sweet	cold, light, dry	PK-, V+
Sweet potato	sweet	cold, heavy, wet	VP-, K+
Taro	sweet, pungent	cold, heavy, wet	PK-, V=
Tomatillo	sour, pungent	hot, light, wet	VK-, P+
Tomato	sweet, sour, pungent	hot, light, wet	VK-, P+
Turnip greens	bitter, pungent	cold, light, dry	PK-, V+
Water chestnut	sweet	cold, light, wet	P-, VK+
Winter melon	sweet	cold, heavy, wet	VP-, K+
Yam (*Dioscorea*)	sweet	cold, heavy, dry	VP-, K+
Yu choy	bitter, pungent	cold, light, dry	PK-, V+
Zucchini	sweet, bitter	cold, light, wet	VP-, K=

Appendix IV: Fruit

Fruit is cold, light and wet in quality, and in general, reduces vata (deficiency) and pitta (inflammation), while potentially increasing kapha (congestion). Fruits that are hot in quality tend to increase digestion (pitta) while decrease kapha (congestion). Fruits that are heavy in quality tend to be difficult to digest, and increase kapha. When dried and cooked, fruit develops more nutritive and restorative properties, suitable to reduce vata. For more information please refer to page 43.

The effect on vata (V), pitta (P) and kapha (K) is noted as an increasing (+), decreasing (-) or neutral (=) effect.

Fruit	Flavor	Quality	Doshas
Açaí	sweet, bitter, sour	cold, heavy, wet	VP-, K=
Acerola	sour, sweet	cold, light, dry	VP, K=
Amla	sour, astringent, sweet	cold, light, dry	VPK-
Apple	sweet, sour	cold, light, wet	PV-, K+
Apricot	sweet, sour	cold, light, wet	VP-, K+
Bael (unripe)	sour	hot, light, wet	VK-, P+
Banana	sweet	cold, heavy, wet	VP-, K+
Bilberry	sweet, sour	cold, light, wet	VP-, K=
Blackberry	sweet, sour	cold, light, wet	VP-, K+
Blueberry	sweet, sour	cold, light, wet	VP-, K=
Breadfruit	sweet	cold, heavy, wet	VP-, K+
Cherry	sweet, sour	cold, light, wet	V-, PK+
Coconut	sweet	cold, heavy, wet	VP-, K+
Cranberry	sour, astringent	cold, light, dry	PK-, V+
Currant	sweet, sour	cold, light, wet	PK-, V+
Date	sweet	cold, heavy, wet	VP-, K+
Durian	sweet	hot, heavy, wet	V-, PK+
Elderberry	sour, bitter, sweet	cold, light, dry	PK-, V+
Fig	sweet	cold, heavy, wet	VP-, K+
Grape	sweet, sour	cold, light, wet	VP-, K+
Grapefruit	sour, sweet	hot, light, wet	K-, VP+
Guava	sweet, sour	cold, light, dry	PK-, V+
Hawthorn	sweet, bitter, sour	hot, light, wet	VK-, P+
Honeydew	sweet	cold, heavy, wet	VP-, K+
Huckleberry	sweet, sour	cold, light, dry	PK-, V+
Kiwi	sweet, sour	cold, light, wet	VP-, K+
Kumquat	sweet, sour	hot, light, wet	VK-, P+
Lemon	sour, bitter	hot, light, wet	KV-, P+

Lime	sour, bitter	hot, light, wet	PK-, V=
Loquat	sweet	cold, heavy, wet	VP-, K+
Lychee	sweet	cold, heavy, wet	V-, KP+
Mango	sweet	cold, heavy, wet	VP-, K+
Mulberry	sweet	cold, light, wet	VP-, K+
Orange (sweet)	sweet, sour	hot, light, wet	VP-, K+
Oregon grape	sour, bitter, sweet	cold, light, dry	PK-, V+
Papaya	sweet	hot, light, wet	VK-, P+
Passionfruit	sweet, sour	cold, light, wet	VP-, K=
Peach	sweet	cold, light, wet	VP-, K+
Pear	sweet	cold, light, wet	VP-, K+
Persimmon	sweet	cold, heavy, wet	VP-, K+
Pineapple	sweet, sour	hot, light, wet	VP-, K+
Pomegranate	sweet, astringent	cold, light, wet	VP-, K=
Pomello	sweet, sour	cold, heavy, wet	VP-, K+
Quince	sour, sweet, astringent	cold, light, dry	PK-, V+
Raspberry	sweet, sour	cold, light, wet	VP-, K=
Rosehip	sour, bitter	cold, light, wet	PK-, V=
Salmonberry	sweet, sour	cold, light, wet	VP-, K=
Strawberry	sweet, sour	cold, light, wet	V-, P+, K=
Tamarind	sour	hot, light, dry	PK-, V=
Thimbleberry	sweet, sour	cold, light, wet	VP-, K=
Watermelon	sweet	cold, heavy, wet	VP-, K+
Wolfberry	sweet	cold, heavy, wet	VP-, K+

Appendix V: Meat

Meat is hot, heavy and wet in quality, and in general, reduces vata (deficiency) while potentially increasing kapha (congestion) and pitta (inflammation). Meat is also difficult to digest, and is best prepared in soups and stews to enhance digestion. For more information please refer to page 45.

The effect on vata (V), pitta (P) and kapha (K) is noted as an increasing (+), decreasing (-) or neutral (=) effect.

Meat	Flavor	Quality	Doshas
Alligator	sweet	hot, heavy, wet	V-, PK+
Anchovy	salty, pungent	hot, light, wet	VK-, P+
Bear	sweet	hot, heavy, wet	V-, PK+
Beef	sweet	hot, heavy, wet	V-, PK+
Bison	sweet	hot, heavy, wet	V-, PK+
Camel	sweet	hot, light, wet	V-, PK+
Chicken	sweet	hot, heavy, wet	VP-, K+
Crab	sweet	cold, heavy, wet	V-, PK+
Crocodile	sweet	hot, heavy, wet	V-, PK+
Deer (venison)	sweet	cold, light, wet	V-, PK=
Duck	sweet	hot, heavy, wet	V-, PK+
Eggs	sweet	hot, heavy, wet	V-, PK+
Frog	sweet	cold, light, wet	VP-, K+
Goat	sweet	hot, light, wet	V-, PK=
Goose	sweet	hot, heavy, wet	V-, PK+
Halibut	sweet, salty	cold, heavy, wet	VP-, K+
Herring	salty, pungent	hot, light, wet	V-, PK+
Horse	sweet, pungent	hot, light, wet	V-, PK+
Iguana	sweet	hot, light, wet	V-, PK=
Lamb	sweet	hot, heavy, wet	V-, PK+
Mackerel	salty, pungent	hot, heavy, wet	V-, PK+
Mutton	sweet	hot, heavy, wet	V-, PK+
Partridge	sweet	cold, light, wet	V-, PK=
Pigeon	sweet	cold, heavy, wet	VP-, K+
Pork	sweet	hot, heavy, wet	V-, PK+
Quail	sweet	hot, light, wet	V-, KP+
Rabbit	sweet	cold, light, wet	PK-, V+
Salmon	sweet, salty	cold, heavy, wet	VP-, K+
Sardine	salty, pungent	hot, light, wet	V-, PK+
Shellfish	sweet, salty	hot, heavy, wet	V-, PK+
Shrimp (prawn)	sweet, salty	hot, light, wet	V-, PK+
Snake	sweet	hot, light, wet	V-, PK+
Trout	sweet	cold, heavy, wet	VP-, K+

Tuna	sweet, salty	hot, heavy, wet	V-, KP+
Turkey	sweet	hot, light, wet	V-, PK+
Turtle	sweet	hot, heavy, wet	VP-, K+
Water buffalo	sweet	hot, heavy, wet	V-, PK+
Yak	sweet	hot, heavy, wet	V-, PK+

Appendix VI: Cereal Grains

Cereal grains are cold, light and dry in quality, and in general, are best for reducing kapha (congestion) and pitta (inflammation). Due to the presence of fiber and antinutrient factors cereal grains are difficult to digest and must prepared according to traditional methods, including germination (p. 116), roasting (p. 121) and fermentation (p. 126). For more information please refer to page 49.

The effect on vata (V), pitta (P) and kapha (K) is noted as an increasing (+), decreasing (-) or neutral (=) effect.

Cereal grains	Flavor	Quality	Doshas
Amaranth	sweet	cold, light, dry	VP-, K=
Barley	sweet, astringent	cold, light, dry	PK-, V=
Buckwheat	sweet, bitter	cold, light, dry	PK-, V=
Coix seed	sweet, pungent	hot, light, dry	K-, VP+
Corn	sweet	cold, light, dry	PK-, V=
Einkorn	sweet	cold, heavy, dry	PV-, K+
Emmer	sweet	cold, heavy, dry	PV-, K+
Finger-Millet	sweet, astringent	cold, light, dry	PK-, V+
Italian Millet	sweet, astringent	cold, light, dry	PK-, V+
Kodo Millet	sweet, astringent	hot, light, dry	PK-, V+
Oat	sweet	cold, heavy, wet	PV-, K+
Proso Millet	sweet, astringent	cold, light, dry	PK-, V+
Quinoa	sweet	cold, light, dry	VP-, K=
Rice	sweet	cold, light, dry	VP-, K=
Rye	sweet, bitter	cold, heavy, wet	VP-, K+
Sawa Millet	sweet, astringent	cold, light, dry	PK-, V+
Sorghum	sweet	cold, light, dry	PK-, V+
Spelt	sweet	cold, heavy, wet	PV-, K+
Teff	sweet	cold, heavy, dry	PV-, K+
Wheat	sweet	cold, heavy, wet	PV-, K+
Wild rice	sweet, bitter	cold, light, dry	PK-, V+

Appendix VII: Legumes

Legumes are cold, light and dry in quality, and in general, are best for reducing kapha (congestion) and pitta (inflammation). Due to the presence of fiber and antinutrient factors legumes are difficult to digest and must prepared according to traditional methods, including germination (p. 116), roasting (p. 121) and fermentation (p. 126). For more information please refer to page 55.

The effect on vata (V), pitta (P) and kapha (K) is noted as an increasing (+), decreasing (-) or neutral (=) effect.

Legume	Flavor	Quality	Doshas
Adzuki bean	sweet, astringent	cold, heavy, dry	PK-, V=
Black-eyed pea	sweet, astringent	cold, heavy, dry	PK-, V+
Chickpea (chana)	sweet, astringent	cold, heavy, dry	PK-, V+
Cowpea	sweet, astringent	cold, heavy, dry	PK-, V+
Fava bean	sweet, astringent	cold, heavy, dry	PK-, V+
Flat bean	sweet, astringent	cold, heavy, dry	PK-, V+
Horse gram	sweet, astringent	cold, heavy, dry	PK-, V+
Kidney bean	sweet, astringent	cold, heavy, dry	PK-, V+
Lentil	sweet, astringent	cold, heavy, dry	PK-, V+
Lima Bean	sweet, astringent	cold, heavy, dry	PK-, V+
Moth bean	sweet, astringent	cold, heavy, dry	PK-, V+
Mung bean	sweet, astringent	cold, heavy, dry	PK-, V=
Pea *(Pisum)*	sweet, astringent	cold, heavy, dry	PK-, V+
Pigeon pea	sweet, astringent	cold, heavy, dry	PK-, V+
Soybeans	sweet, astringent	cold, heavy, dry	PK-, V+
Urad bean	sweet, astringent	hot, heavy, dry	V-, PK+

Appendix VIII: Nuts and Seeds

Nuts and seeds are hot, heavy and wet in quality, and due to the presence of antinutrient factors can be difficult to digest. In general, nuts and seeds are useful to counter vata (deficiency), but may increase pitta (inflammation) and kapha (congestion). Nuts listed below are all assumed to be fresh, and not rancid, which results in a distinct bitter flavor. For more information please refer to page 58.

The effect on vata (V), pitta (P) and kapha (K) is noted as an increasing (+), decreasing (-) or neutral (=) effect.

Nuts and seeds	Flavor	Quality	Doshas
Almond	sweet	hot, heavy, wet	V-, PK+
Coconut	sweet	cold, heavy, wet	VP-, K+
Cashew	sweet	hot, heavy, wet	VP-, K+
Chestnut	sweet	hot, heavy, wet	VP-, K+
Pinenut	sweet	hot, light, wet	V-, KP+
Pecan	sweet	hot, heavy, wet	VP-, K+
Walnut	sweet	hot, heavy, wet	V-, PK+
Hazelnut	sweet	hot, light, wet	V-, PK+
Pumpkin seed	sweet, bitter	hot, heavy, wet	VK-, P+
Sesame seed	sweet, bitter	hot, heavy, wet	V-, PK+
Sunflower seed	sweet	cold, light, wet	V-, PK+
Hemp seed	sweet	hot, heavy, wet	V-, PK+
Flax seed	sweet, bitter	hot, heavy, wet	V-, PK+
Peanut	sweet	hot, heavy, wet	V-, PK+

Appendix IX: Dairy Products

Dairy foods and beverages are generally cool, heavy and wet in nature, and tend to decrease vata (deficiency) and pitta (inflammation), but increase kapha (congestion). For more information please refer to page 61.

The effect on vata (V), pitta (P) and kapha (K) is noted as an increasing (+), decreasing (-) or neutral (=) effect.

Dairy product	Flavor	Quality	Doshas
Aged cheese	sweet, pungent	cold, heavy, dry	V-, PK+
Boiled milk	sweet	hot, light, wet	VP-, K=
Butter (cultured)	sweet, sour	cold, heavy, wet	VP-, K+
Buttermilk	sour, sweet	cold, light, wet	VP-, K+
Ghee	sweet	cold, heavy, wet	VP-, K+
Kefir	sour, sweet	hot, heavy, wet	V-, PK+
Panir	sweet	cold, heavy, wet	VP-, K+
Raw milk	sweet	cold, heavy, wet	VP-, K+
Yogurt	sour	hot, heavy, wet	V-, PK+

Appendix X: Fats and Oils

Fats and oils are generally hot, heavy and wet in nature, and tend to decrease vata (deficiency) and pitta (inflammation), but may increase kapha (congestion). For more information please refer to page 67.

The effect on vata (V), pitta (P) and kapha (K) is noted as an increasing (+), decreasing (-) or neutral (=) effect.

Fats and oils	Flavor	Quality	Doshas
Almond oil	sweet	hot, heavy, wet	V-, PK+
Canola oil	sweet, pungent	hot, light, wet	VPK+
Castor oil	sweet, pungent	hot, heavy, wet	V-, PK+
Coco butter	sweet	cold, heavy, wet	VP-, K+
Coconut oil	sweet	cold, heavy, wet	VP-, K+
Fish oil	sweet, salty, pungent	hot, heavy, wet	VP-, K+
Flax oil	sweet, bitter	hot, heavy, wet	V-, PK+
Ghee	sweet	cold, heavy, wet	VP-, K+
Hazelnut oil	sweet	hot, heavy, wet	V-, PK+
Hemp oil	sweet	hot, heavy, wet	V-, PK+
Lard/tallow oil	sweet	hot, heavy, wet	V-, PK+
Mustard oil	sweet, pungent	hot, light wet	VK-, P+
Olive oil	sweet	hot, heavy, wet	VP-, K+
Peanut oil	sweet	hot, heavy, wet	V-, PK+
Safflower oil	sweet	hot, heavy, wet	V-, PK+
Sunflower oil	sweet	hot, heavy, wet	V-, PK+
Walnut oil	sweet	hot, heavy, wet	V-, PK+

References

[1] Starfield B. 2000. Is US health really the best in the world? *JAMA*. 284(4):483-5.

[2] Duhigg C. "Millions in U.S. Drink Dirty Water, Records Show," New York Times 7 Dec 2009. Available from: http://www.nytimes.com/2009/12/08/business/energy-environment/08water.html?_r=1

[3] Huang AT, Batterman S. 2009. Formation of trihalomethanes in foods and beverages. *Food Addit Contam Part A Chem Anal Control Expo Risk Assess*. 26(7):947-57.

[4] Connett P, Beck J, Micklem HS. 2010. *The Case Against Fluoride*. Chelsea Green: White River Junction VA

[5] Michels HT, Noyce JO, Keevil CW. 2009. Effects of temperature and humidity on the efficacy of methicillin-resistant *Staphylococcus aureus* challenged antimicrobial materials containing silver and copper. *Lett Appl Microbiol*. 49(2):191-5

[6] Martín-Domíngueza A, Alarcón-Herrerab MT, Martín-Domínguezb IR, González-Herrerac A. 2005. Efficiency in the disinfection of water for human consumption in rural communities using solar radiation. *Solar Energy* 78(1):31-40

[7] Klonoff DC. 2009. The beneficial effects of a Paleolithic diet on type 2 diabetes and other risk factors for cardiovascular disease. *J Diabetes Sci Technol*. 3(6):1229-32.

[8] Clifton PM, Bastiaans K, Keogh JB. 2009. High protein diets decrease total and abdominal fat and improve CVD risk profile in overweight and obese men and women with elevated triacylglycerol. *Nutr Metab Cardiovasc Dis*. 19(8):548-54

[9] Zhou W, Mukherjee P, Kiebish MA, Markis WT, Mantis JG, Seyfried TN. 2007. The calorically restricted ketogenic diet, an effective alternative therapy for malignant brain cancer. *Nutr Metab (Lond)*. 4:5.

[10] Reaven GM. 2005. Insulin resistance, the insulin resistance syndrome, and cardiovascular disease. *Panminerva Med*. 47(4):201-10.

[11] Donaldson SG, Van Oostdam J, Tikhonov C, Feeley M, Armstrong B, Ayotte P, Boucher O, Bowers W, Chan L, Dallaire F, Dallaire R, Dewailly E, Edwards J, Egeland GM, Fontaine J, Furgal C, Leech T, Loring E, Muckle G, Nancarrow T, Pereg D, Plusquellec P, Potyrala M, Receveur O, Shearer RG. 2010. Environmental contaminants and human health in the Canadian Arctic. *Sci Total Environ*. 408(22):5165-234

[12] Ohta S, Ishizuka D, Nishimura H, Nakao T, Aozasa O, Shimidzu Y, Ochiai F, Kida T, Nishi M, Miyata H. 2002. Comparison of polybrominated diphenyl ethers in fish, vegetables, and meats and levels in human milk of nursing women in Japan. *Chemosphere*. 46(5):689-96.

[13] Norén K. 1983. Levels of organochlorine contaminants in human milk in relation to the dietary habits of the mothers. *Acta Paediatr Scand*. 72(6):811-6.

[14] Fraser AJ, Webster TF, McClean MD. 2009. Diet contributes significantly to the body burden of PBDEs in the general U.S. population. *Environ Health Perspect.*117(10):1520-5

[15] Dickman MD, Leung CK, Leong MK. 1998. Hong Kong male subfertility links to mercury in human hair and fish. *Sci Total Environ.* 214:165-74.

[16] Jones-Otazo HA, Clarke JP, Diamond ML, Archbold JA, Ferguson G, Harner T, Richardson GM, Ryan JJ, Wilford B. 2005. Is house dust the missing exposure pathway for PBDEs? An analysis of the urban fate and human exposure to PBDEs. *Environ Sci Technol.* 39(14):5121-30.

[17] Johnson-Restrepo B, Kannan K. 2009. An assessment of sources and pathways of human exposure to polybrominated diphenyl ethers in the United States. *Chemosphere.* 76(4):542-8.

[18] Van Audenhaege M, Heraud F, Menard C, Bouyrie J, Morois S, Calamassi-Tran G, Lesterle S, Volatier JL, Leblanc JC. 2009. Impact of food consumption habits on the pesticide dietary intake: Comparison between a French vegetarian and the general population. *Food Addit Contam Part A Chem Anal Control Expo Risk Assess.* 26(10):1372-88.

[19] Schecter A, Harris TR, Päpke O, Tung KC, Musumba A. 2006. Polybrominated diphenyl ether (PBDE) levels in the blood of pure vegetarians (vegans). *Toxicol Environ Chem.* 88: 1, 107-12

[20] Health Canada. 2002. Fish and Seafood Survey. Available from: http://www.hc-sc.gc.ca/fn-an/surveill/other-autre/fish-poisson/index-eng.php

[21] Health Canada. 2008. Mercury in Fish – Questions and Answers. Available from: http://www.hc-sc.gc.ca/fn-an/securit/chem-chim/environ/mercur/merc_fish_qa-poisson_qr-eng.php

[22] Cordain L. 1999. Cereal grains: humanity's double-edged sword. *World Rev Nutr Diet.* 84:19-73

[23] Sanders, LJ. 2002. From Thebes to Toronto and the 21st Century: An Incredible Journey. *Diabetes Spectrum* 15(1): 56-60

[24] Young TK, Reading J, Elias B, O'Neil JD. 2000. Type 2 diabetes mellitus in Canada's first nations: status of an epidemic in progress. *CMAJ.* 163(5):561-6.

[25] Reaven GM. 2005. Insulin resistance, the insulin resistance syndrome, and cardiovascular disease. *Panminerva Med.* 47(4):201-10

[26] Anderson JW, Baird P, Davis RH Jr, Ferreri S, Knudtson M, Koraym A, Waters V, Williams CL. 2009. Health benefits of dietary fiber. *Nutr Rev.* 67(4):188-205.

[27] Miyake K, Tanaka T, McNeil PL. 2007. Lectin-based food poisoning: a new mechanism of protein toxicity. *PLoS One.* 2(1):e687

[28] Cordain L, Toohey L, Smith MJ, Hickey MS. 2000. Modulation of immune function by dietary lectins in rheumatoid arthritis. *Br J Nutr.* 83(3):207-17

[29] Ryder SD, Parker N, Ecclestone D, Haqqani MT, Rhodes JM. 1994. Peanut lectin stimulates proliferation in colonic explants from patients with inflammatory bowel disease and colon polyps. *Gastroenterology.* 106(1):117-24

[30] Harrison MS, Wehbi M, Obideen K. 2007. Celiac disease: more common than you think. *Cleve Clin J Med.* 74(3):209-15.

[31] Fine K. 2003. Early Diagnosis Of Gluten Sensitivity: Before the Villi are Gone. Available from http://www.finerhealth.com/Essay

[32] Nelsen DA Jr. 2002. Gluten-sensitive enteropathy (celiac disease): more common than you think. *Am Fam Physician.* 66(12):2259-66.

[33] Ibid.

[34] Ibid.

[35] Ibid.

[36] Birkenfeld S, Dreiher J, Weitzman D, Cohen AD. 2009. Coeliac disease associated with psoriasis. *Br J Dermatol.* 161(6):1331-4.

[37] Ch'ng CL, Jones MK, Kingham JG. 2007. Celiac disease and autoimmune thyroid disease. *Clin Med Res.* 5(3):184-92.

[38] Bhadada SK, Kochhar R, Bhansali A, Dutta U, Kumar PR, Poornachandra KS, Vaiphei K, Nain CK, Singh K. 2011. Prevalence and clinical profile of celiac disease in type 1 diabetes mellitus in north India. *J Gastroenterol Hepatol.* 26(2):378-381.

[39] Krifa F, Knani L, Sakly W, Ghedira I, Essoussi AS, Boukadida J, Ben Hadj Hamida F. 2010. Uveitis responding on gluten free diet in a girl with celiac disease and diabetes mellitus type 1. *Gastroenterol Clin Biol.* 34(4-5):319-20.

[40] Elfström P, Montgomery SM, Kämpe O, Ekbom A, Ludvigsson JF. 2007. Risk of primary adrenal insufficiency in patients with celiac disease. *J. Clin. End. & Metab.* 92(9): 3595

[41] Collin P, Vilska S, Heinonen PK, Hällström O, Pikkarainen P. 1996. Infertility and coeliac disease. *Gut.* 39(3):382–4.

[42] Leeds JS, Höroldt BS, Sidhu R, et al. 2007. Is there an association between coeliac disease and inflammatory bowel diseases? A study of relative prevalence in comparison with population controls. *Scand. J. Gastroenterol.* 42(10):1214–20

[43] Niveloni S, Dezi R, Pedreira S, Podestá A, Cabanne A, Vazquez H, Sugai E, Smecuol E, Doldan I, Valero J, Kogan Z, Boerr L, Mauriño E, Terg R, Bai JC. 1998. Gluten sensitivity in patients with primary biliary cirrhosis. *Am J Gastroenterol.* 93(3):404-8.

[44] Volta U, Rodrigo L, Granito A, et al. 2002. Celiac disease in autoimmune cholestatic liver disorders. *Am. J. Gastroenterol.* 97(10):2609–13

[45] Patel RS, Johlin FC, Murray JA. 1999. Celiac disease and recurrent pancreatitis. *Gastrointest. Endosc.* 50(6): 823–7

[46] Hadjivassiliou M, Rao DG, Wharton SB, Sanders DS, Grünewald RA, Davies-Jones AG. 2010. Sensory ganglionopathy due to gluten sensitivity. *Neurology.* 75(11):1003-8.

[47] Hu WT, Murray JA, Greenaway MC, Parisi JE, Josephs KA. 2006. Cognitive impairment and celiac disease. *Arch Neurol.* 63(10):1440-6.

[48] Canales P, Mery VP, Larrondo FJ, Bravo FL, Godoy J. 2006. Epilepsy and celiac disease: favorable outcome with a gluten-free diet in a patient refractory to antiepileptic drugs. *Neurologist.* 12(6):318-21.

[49] Mavroudi A, Karatza E, Papastavrou T, Panteliadis C, Spiroglou K. 2005. Successful treatment of epilepsy and celiac disease with a gluten-free diet. *Pediatr Neurol.* 33(4):292-5.

[50] Addolorato G, Capristo E, Ghittoni G, et al. 2001. Anxiety but not depression decreases in coeliac patients after one-year gluten-free diet: a longitudinal study. *Scand. J. Gastroenterol.* 36(5): 502–6

[51] Gabrielli M, Cremonini F, Fiore G, Addolorato G, Padalino C, Candelli M, De Leo ME, Santarelli L, Giacovazzo M, Gasbarrini A, Pola P, Gasbarrini A. 2003. Association between migraine and Celiac disease: results from a preliminary case-control and therapeutic study. *Am J Gastroenterol.* 98(3):625-9.

[52] Wallace DJ, Hallegua DS. 2004. Fibromyalgia: the gastrointestinal link. *Curr Pain Headache Rep.* 8(5):364-8.

[53] Sökjer M, Jónsson T, Bödvarsson S, Jónsdóttir I, Valdimarsson H. 1995. Selective increase of IgA rheumatoid factor in patients with gluten sensitivity. *Acta Derm Venereol.* 75(2): 130–2

[54] Al-Mayouf SM, Al-Mehaidib AI, Alkaff MA. 2003. The significance of elevated serologic markers of celiac disease in children with juvenile rheumatoid arthritis. *Saudi J Gastroenterol.* 9(2):75-8.

[55] Kemppainen T, Kröger H, Janatuinen E, Arnala I, Kosma VM, Pikkarainen P, Julkunen R, Jurvelin J, Alhava E, Uusitupa M. 1999. Osteoporosis in adult patients with celiac disease. *Bone.* 24(3):249-55.

[56] Holmes GK, Stokes PL, Sorahan TM, Prior P, Waterhouse JA, Cooke WT. 1976. Coeliac disease, gluten-free diet, and malignancy. *Gut.* 17(8): 612–9

[57] Ferguson A, Kingstone K. 1996. Coeliac disease and malignancies. *Acta Paediatr Suppl.* 412:78-81.

[58] Häuser W, Janke KH, Klump B, Gregor M, Hinz A. 2010. Anxiety and depression in adult patients with celiac disease on a gluten-free diet. *World J Gastroenterol.* 16(22):2780-7.

[59] De Angelis M, Cassone A, Rizzello CG, Gagliardi F, Minervini F, Calasso M, Di Cagno R, Francavilla R, Gobbetti M. 2010. Mechanism of degradation of immunogenic gluten epitopes from Triticum turgidum L. var. durum by sourdough lactobacilli and fungal proteases. *Appl Environ Microbiol.* 76(2):508-18.

[60] Di Cagno R, De Angelis M, Auricchio S, Greco L, Clarke C, De Vincenzi M, Giovannini C, D'Archivio M, Landolfo F, Parrilli G, Minervini F, Arendt E, Gobbetti M. 2004. Sourdough bread made from wheat and nontoxic flours and started with selected lactobacilli is tolerated in celiac sprue patients. *Appl Environ Microbiol.* 70(2):1088-96.

[61] Yan L, Spitznagel EL. 2005. Meta-analysis of soy food and risk of prostate cancer in men. *Int J Cancer.* 117(4):667-9

[62] Tong X, Li W, Qin LQ. 2010. Meta-analysis of the relationship between soybean product consumption and gastric cancer. *Zhonghua Yu Fang Yi Xue Za Zhi.* 44(3):215-20.

[63] Yan L, Spitznagel EL, Bosland MC. 2010. Soy consumption and colorectal cancer risk in humans: a meta-analysis. *Cancer Epidemiol Biomarkers Prev.* 19(1):148-58

[64] Carmignani LO, Pedro AO, Costa-Paiva LH, Pinto-Neto AM. 2010. The effect of dietary soy supplementation compared to estrogen and placebo on menopausal symptoms: a randomized controlled trial. *Maturitas.* 67(3):262-9.

[65] Enneking D, Wink M. 2000. "Towards the elimination of anti-nutritional factors in grain legumes," In: *Linking Research and Marketing Opportunities for Pulses in the 21st Century.* Norwell MA: Kluwer Academic. p 671-83

[66] Copper J, Bloom FE, Roth RH. 1996. *The Biochemical Basis of Neuropharmacology.* New York: Oxford University Press p. 188

[67] Chien HL, Huang HY, Chou CC. 2006. Transformation of isoflavone phytoestrogens during the fermentation of soymilk with lactic acid bacteria and bifidobacteria. *Food Microbiol.* 23(8):772-8.

[68] Chang TS, Ding HY, Tai SS, Wu CY. 2007. Metabolism of the soy isoflavones daidzein and genistein by fungi used in the preparation of various fermented soybean foods. *Biosci Biotechnol Biochem.* 71(5):1330-3.

[69] Okabe Y, Shimazu T, Tanimoto H. 2010. Higher bioavailability of isoflavones after a single ingestion of aglycone-rich fermented soybeans compared with glucoside-rich non-fermented soybeans in Japanese postmenopausal women. *J Sci Food Agric.* Nov 22. [Epub ahead of print]

[70] White et al 2000. Brain Aging and Midlife Tofu Consumption. *Journal of the American College of Nutrition,* 19(2):242-255

[71] Cederroth et al. 2010. Soy, phyto-oestrogens and male reproductive function: a review. *Int J Androl.* 33(2):304-16

[72] Jefferson WN, Padilla-Banks E, Newbold RR. 2007. Disruption of the female reproductive system by the phytoestrogen genistein. *Reprod Toxicol.* 23(3):308-16

[73] Chandrareddy A, Muneyyirci-Delale O, McFarlane SI, Murad OM. 2008. Adverse effects of phytoestrogens on reproductive health: a report of three cases. *Complement Ther Clin Pract.* 14(2):132-5

[74] Helferich WG, Andrade JE, Hoagland MS. 2008. Phytoestrogens and breast cancer: a complex story. *Inflammopharmacology.* 16(5):219-26

[75] Dave B, Wynne R, Su Y, Korourian S, Chang JC, Simmen RC. 2010. Enhanced mammary progesterone receptor-A isoform activity in the promotion of mammary tumor progression by dietary soy in rats. *Nutr Cancer.* 62(6):774-82.

[76] Park JW, Kim YB. 2006. Effect of pressure cooking on aflatoxin B1 in rice. *J Agric Food Chem.* 54(6):2431-5

[77] Salah E, Mahgoub O, Safia A, Elhag. 1988. Effect of milling, soaking, malting, heat-treatment and fermentation on phytate level of four Sudanese sorghum cultivars. *Food Chemistry.* 61(1-2):77-80

[78] Duhan, A., Chauhan, B. M., Punia, D. and Kapoor, A. C. 1989. Phytic acid content of chickpea (*Cicer arietinum*) and black gram (*Vigna mungo*): varietal differences and effect of domestic processing and cooking methods. *Journal of the Science of Food and Agriculture.* 49:449–455.

[79] Mbithi-Mwikya S, Van Camp J, Yiru Y, Huyghebaert A. 2000. Nutrient and Antinutrient Changes in Finger Millet (Eleusine coracan) During Sprouting, Lebensmittel-*Wissenschaft und-Technologie.* 33(1):9-14

[80] Armbrecht HJ, Wasserman RH. 1976. Enhancement of Ca++ uptake by lactose in the rat small intestine. *J Nutr* 106(9):1265-71.

[81] Melnik BC. 2009. Milk: the promoter of chronic Western diseases. *Med Hypotheses* Jun;72(6):631-9.

[82] Chan JM, Gann PH, Giovannucci EL. 2005. Role of diet in prostate cancer development and progression. *J Clin Oncol.* 23(32):8152-60.

[83] Vaarala, O. et al. 1999. Cow's milk formula feeding induces primary immunization to insulin in infants at genetic risk for type 1 diabetes. *Diabetes*. Jul; 48(7):1389-94

[84] Roth-Walter F, Berin MC, Arnaboldi P, Escalante CR, Dahan S, Rauch J, Jensen-Jarolim E, Mayer L. 2008. Pasteurization of milk proteins promotes allergic sensitization by enhancing uptake through Peyer's patches. *Allergy*. 63(7):882-90.

[85] Krauss WE, Erb JH, Washburn RG. 1933. Studies on the nutritive value of milk, II. The effect of pasteurization on some of the nutritive properties of milk. *Ohio Agricultural Experiment Station Bulletin*. 518:7

[86] Rolls BA, Porter JW. 1973. Some effects of processing and storage on the nutritive value of milk and milk products. *Proc Nutr Soc*. 32(1):9-15.

[87] Gregory JF. 1982. Denaturation of the folacin-binding protein in pasteurized milk products. *J Nutr*. 112(7):1329-38

[88] Ranieri ML, Boor KJ. 2009. Short communication: bacterial ecology of high-temperature, short-time pasteurized milk processed in the United States. *J Dairy Sci*. 92(10):4833-40.

[89] Ranieri ML, Huck JR, Sonnen M, Barbano DM, Boor KJ. 2009. High temperature, short time pasteurization temperatures inversely affect bacterial numbers during refrigerated storage of pasteurized fluid milk. *J Dairy Sci*. 92(10):4823-32.

[90] Ouyang J, Pei Z, Lutwick L, Dalal S, Yang L, Cassai N, Sandhu K, Hanna B, Wieczorek RL, Bluth M, Pincus MR. 2008. Case report: *Paenibacillus thiaminolyticus*: a new cause of human infection, inducing bacteremia in a patient on hemodialysis. *Ann Clin Lab Sci*. 38(4):393-400.

[91] Rank P. 1986. Milk and arteriosclerosis. *Med Hypotheses*. 20(3):317-38.

[92] Goff D. 2010. 'Homogenization of Milk and Milk Products', Dairy Science and Technology, University of Guelph. Available from: http://www.foodsci.uoguelph.ca/dairyedu/homogenization.html

[93] Kirn TF. 2004. Prevalence of cow's milk allergy continues to rise: caution urged for challenge testing. *Family Practice News*. April 01

[94] Srikanthamurthy, KR. 2001. *Bhavaprakasha of Bhavamishra*. Varanasi: Krishnadas Academy, p. 455

[95] Bell SJ, Grochoski GT, Clarke AJ. 2006. Health implications of milk containing beta-casein with the A2 genetic variant. *Crit Rev Food Sci Nutr*. 46(1):93-100.

[96] Slots T, Butler G, Leifert C, Kristensen T, Skibsted LH, Nielsen JH. 2009. Potentials to differentiate milk composition by different feeding strategies. *J Dairy Sci*. 92(5):2057-66.

[97] Simopoulos AP. 2008. The importance of the omega-6/omega-3 fatty acid ratio in cardiovascular disease and other chronic diseases. *Exp Biol Med* (Maywood). 233(6):674-88

[98] Lafarge V, Ogier JC, Girard V, Maladen V, Leveau JY, Gruss A, Delacroix-Buchet A. 2004. Raw cow milk bacterial population shifts attributable to refrigeration. *Appl Environ Microbiol*. 70(9):5644-50

[99] Heuvelink AE, van Heerwaarden C, Zwartkruis-Nahuis A, Tilburg JJ, Bos MH, Heilmann FG, Hofhuis A, Hoekstra T, de Boer E. 2009. Two outbreaks of

campylobacteriosis associated with the consumption of raw cows' milk. *Int J Food Microbiol.* 134(1-2):70-4.

[100] Oliver SP, Boor KJ, Murphy SC, Murinda SE. 2009. Food safety hazards associated with consumption of raw milk. *Foodborne Pathog Dis.* 6(7):793-806.

[101] Guh A, Phan Q, Nelson R, Purviance K, Milardo E, Kinney S, Mshar P, Kasacek W, Cartter M. 2008. Outbreak of Escherichia coli O157 associated with raw milk, Connecticut, 2008. *Clin Infect Dis.* 51(12):1411-7.

[102] Dash, B. 1991. *Materia Medica of Ayurveda.* New Delhi: B. Jain Publishers, p. 390-91

[103] Yang W, Lu J, Weng J, Jia W, Ji L, Xiao J, Shan Z, Liu J, Tian H, Ji Q, Zhu D, Ge J, Lin L, Chen L, Guo X, Zhao Z, Li Q, Zhou Z, Shan G, He J. 2010. Prevalence of diabetes among men and women in China. *N Engl J Med.* 362(12):1090-101.

[104] Cow butterfat also contains 2.9% butyric acid (4:0).

[105] Goat butterfat contains 2.2% butyric acid (4:0), 2.5% caproic acid (6:0) and 2.8% caprylic acid (8:0).

[106] Leray C. 2010. Cyperlipid Center: Resource site for lipid studies. Available from: http://www.cyberlipid.org/cyberlip/home0001.htm

[107] Kiralan M, Gul V, Metin Kara S. 2010. Fatty acid composition of hempseed oils from different locations in Turkey. *SJAR.* 8(2):385-90

[108] Simopoulos AP. 2008. The importance of the omega-6/omega-3 fatty acid ratio in cardiovascular disease and other chronic diseases. *Exp Biol Med (Maywood).* 233(6):674-88

[109] Simopoulos AP. 2006. Evolutionary aspects of diet, the omega-6/omega-3 ratio and genetic variation: nutritional implications for chronic diseases. *Biomed Pharmacother.* 60(9):502-7.

[110] "We have found in our laboratories at NDSU (Pizzey and Hall III, unpublished data) that hexane extracted flaxseed oil oxidized relatively quickly under slightly elevated temperatures (40°C) and in the presence of sunlight. Compared to freshly extracted oil, samples stored under sunlight had a 200 fold increase in peroxide values within 12 days while samples stored in the dark at 40°C had peroxide values 50 fold higher by day 12." Available from: http://www.ameriflax.com/default.cfm?page=flax_ndsu

[111] Mozaffarian D, Cao H, King IB, Lemaitre RN, Song X, Siscovick DS, Hotamisligil GS. 2010. Trans-palmitoleic Acid, metabolic risk factors, and new-onset diabetes in US adults: a cohort study. *Ann Intern Med.* 153(12):790-9

[112] Godwin A, Prabhu R. 2006. Lipid peroxidation of fish oils. *Indian Journal of Clinical Biochemistry.* 21(1):202-204

[113] Wolff R. 1993. Further Studies on Artificial Geometrical Isomers of a-Linolenic Acid in Edible Linolenic Acid-Containing Oils. *JAOCS* 70(3):219-224

[114] Prabhu HR. 2000. Lipid peroxidation in culinary oils subjected to thermal stress. *Indian Journal of Clinical Biochemistry.* 15(1):1-5

[115] Bernstein, Richard. 1997. *Dr. Bernstein's Diabetes Solution.* New York: Little Brown and Company, p. 318

[116] EFSA Panel on Biological Hazards (BIOHAZ). 2010. Scientific Opinion on Fish Oil for Human Consumption. Food Hygiene, including Rancidity. *EFSA*

Journal. 8(10):1874. Available online:
http://www.efsa.europa.eu/en/efsajournal/scdoc/1874.htm

[117] Pak CS. 2005. Stability and quality of fish oil during domestic application. The United Nations University, Fisheries Training Program. Unpublished thesis. Available from: www.unuftp.is/static/fellows/document/pak05prf.pdf

[118] Fritsche KL, Johnston PV. 1988. Rapid autoxidation of fish oil in diets without added antioxidants. *J Nutr.* 118(4):425-6

[119] Colantuoni C, Rada P, McCarthy J, Patten C, Avena NM, Chadeayne A, Hoebel BG. 2002. Evidence that intermittent, excessive sugar intake causes endogenous opioid dependence. *Obes Res.* 10(6):478-88.

[120] Soffritti M, Belpoggi F, Manservigi M, Tibaldi E, Lauriola M, Falcioni L, Bua L. 2010. Aspartame administered in feed, beginning prenatally through life span, induces cancers of the liver and lung in male Swiss mice. *Am J Ind Med.* 53(12):1197-206

[121] Karstadt M. 2010. Inadequate toxicity tests of food additive acesulfame. *Int J Occup Environ Health.* 16(1):89-96

[122] Humphries P, Pretorius E, Naudé H. 2008. Direct and indirect cellular effects of aspartame on the brain. *Eur J Clin Nutr.* 62(4):451-62.

[123] Swithers SE, Martin AA, Davidson TL. 2010. High-intensity sweeteners and energy balance. *Physiol Behav.* 100(1):55-62

[124] USDA. Agriculture Research Service. Dr. Duke's Phytochemical and Ethnobotanical Databases. [Online Database] 15 February 2011. Available from: http://www.ars-grin.gov/duke/

[125] Food Services Agency. 2004. Survey of caffeine levels in hot beverages. Available from: http://www.food.gov.uk/multimedia/pdfs/fsis5304.pdf

[126] USDA. Agriculture Research Service. Dr. Duke's Phytochemical and Ethnobotanical Databases. [Online Database] 15 February 2011. Available from: http://www.ars-grin.gov/duke/

[127] Kimura K, Ozeki M, Juneja LR, Ohira H. 2007. L-Theanine reduces psychological and physiological stress responses. *Biol Psychol.* 74(1):39-45.

[128] Lambert JD, Elias RJ. 2010. The antioxidant and pro-oxidant activities of green tea polyphenols: a role in cancer prevention. *Arch Biochem Biophys.* 501(1):65-72

[129] Suganuma M, Saha A, Fujiki H. 2011. New cancer treatment strategy using combination of green tea catechins and anticancer drugs. *Cancer Sci.* 102(2):317-23.

[130] Kuriyama S, Shimazu T, Ohmori K, Kikuchi N, Nakaya N, Nishino Y, Tsubono Y, Tsuji I. 2006. Green tea consumption and mortality due to cardiovascular disease, cancer, and all causes in Japan: the Ohsaki study. *JAMA.* 296(10):1255-65.

[131] Wong MH, Fung KF, Carr HP. 2003. Aluminium and fluoride contents of tea, with emphasis on brick tea and their health implications. *Toxicol Lett.* 137(1-2):111-20.

[132] Lung SC, Cheng HW, Fu CB. 2008. Potential exposure and risk of fluoride intakes from tea drinks produced in Taiwan. *J Expo Sci Environ Epidemiol.* 18(2):158-66.

[133] di Tomaso E, Beltramo M, Piomelli D. 1996. Brain cannabinoids in chocolate. *Nature*. 382(6593):677-8

[134] Ziegleder G, Stojacic E, Stumpf B. 1992. Occurrence of beta-phenylethylamine and its derivatives in cocoa and cocoa products. *Z Lebensm Unters Forsch*. 195(3):235-8

[135] Herraiz T. 2000. Tetrahydro-beta-carbolines, potential neuroactive alkaloids, in chocolate and cocoa. *J Agric Food Chem*. 48(10):4900-4.

[136] Strandberg TE, Strandberg AY, Pitkälä K, Salomaa VV, Tilvis RS, Miettinen TA. 2007. Chocolate, well-being and health among elderly men. *Eur J Clin Nutr*. 62(2):247-53.

[137] Parker G, Crawford J. 2007. Chocolate craving when depressed: a personality marker. *Br J Psychiatry*. 191:351-2.

[138] Messaoudi M, Bisson JF, Nejdi A, Rozan P, Javelot H. 2008. Antidepressant-like effects of a cocoa polyphenolic extract in Wistar-Unilever rats. *Nutr Neurosci*. 11(6):269-76

[139] Steinberg FM, Bearden MM, Keen CL. 2003. Cocoa and chocolate flavonoids: implications for cardiovascular health. *J Am Diet Assoc*. 103(2):215-23.

[140] Selmi C, Mao TK, Keen CL, Schmitz HH, Eric Gershwin M. 2006. The anti-inflammatory properties of cocoa flavanols. *J Cardiovasc Pharmacol*. 47 Suppl 2:S163-71

[141] Erdman JW Jr, Carson L, Kwik-Uribe C, Evans EM, Allen RR. 2008. Effects of cocoa flavanols on risk factors for cardiovascular disease. *Asia Pac J Clin Nutr*. 17 Suppl 1:284-7.

[142] K Hollenberg N. 2006. Vascular action of cocoa flavanols in humans: the roots of the story. *J Cardiovasc Pharmacol*. 47 Suppl 2:S99-102

[143] Patel AK, Rogers JT, Huang X. 2008. Flavanols, mild cognitive impairment, and Alzheimer's dementia. *Int J Clin Exp Med*. 1(2):181-91

[144] Aremu CY, Agiang MA, Ayatse JO. 1995. Nutrient and antinutrient profiles of raw and fermented cocoa beans. *Plant Foods Hum Nutr*. 48(3):217-23.

[145] Sánchez-Hervás M, Gil JV, Bisbal F, Ramón D, Martínez-Culebras PV. 2008. Mycobiota and mycotoxin producing fungi from cocoa beans. *Int J Food Microbiol*. 125(3):336-40.

[146] Weinberg BA, Bealer BK. 2001. *The world of caffeine: the science and culture of the world's most popular drug*. New York: Rutledge, p. 10-12

[147] FAO. 2003. '4. Sugar and Beverages', in Agricultural Commodities: Profiles And Relevant WTO Negotiating Issues. Available from: www.fao.org/docrep/006/y4343e/y4343e05.htm

[148] USDA. Agriculture Research Service. Dr. Duke's Phytochemical and Ethnobotanical Databases. [Online Database] 16 February 2011. Available from: http://www.ars-grin.gov/duke/

[149] McCusker RR, Goldberger BA, Cone EJ. 2003. Caffeine content of specialty coffees. *J Anal Toxicol*. 27(7):520-2.

[150] USDA. 2010. USDA National Nutrient Database for Standard Reference, Release 23. Available from: www.nal.usda.gov/fnic/foodcomp/search/

[151] Weinberg BA, Bealer BK. 2001. *The world of caffeine: the science and culture of the world's most popular drug*. New York: Rutledge, p. 6-7

[152] USDA. Agriculture Research Service. Dr. Duke's Phytochemical and Ethnobotanical Databases. [Online Database] 16 February 2011. Available from: http://www.ars-grin.gov/duke/

[153] Cikitsa sthana VII:87

[154] Milligan SR, Kalita JC, Heyerick A, Rong H, De Cooman L, De Keukeleire D. 1999. Identification of a potent phytoestrogen in hops (*Humulus lupulus* L.) and beer. *J Clin Endocrinol Metab*. 84(6):2249-52.

[155] Carmody RN, Wrangham RW. 2009. The energetic significance of cooking. *J Hum Evol*. 57(4):379-91.

[156] Carmody RN, Wrangham RW. 2009. Cooking and the human commitment to a high-quality diet. *Cold Spring Harb Symp Quant Biol*. 74:427-34

[157] Cordain L, Miller JB, Eaton SB, Mann N, Holt SHA, Speth JD. 2000. Plant-animal subsistence ratios and macronutrient energy estimations in worldwide hunter-gatherer diets. *Am J Clin Nutr*. 71:682–92

[158] Trowell HHC, Burkitt DP. 1981. *Western Diseases: Their Emergence and Prevention*. Cambridge MA: Harvard University Press

[159] Wild S, Roglic G, Green A, Sicree R, King H. 2004. Global prevalence of diabetes: estimates for the year 2000 and projections for 2030. *Diabetes Care*. 27(5):1047-53

[160] Gurven M, Kaplan H. 2003. Longevity Among Hunter-Gatherers: A Cross Cultural Examination. *Population and Development Review* 33(2):321-365

[161] Truswell AS. 1977. Diet and nutrition of hunter-gatherers. *Ciba Found Symp*. (49):213-21

[162] Neel JV. 1977. Health and disease in unacculturated Amerindian populations. *Ciba Found Symp*. (49):155-68

[163] Montaigne ML. 1886. *The Essayes of Michael Lord of Montaigne*. Translated by John Florio, edited by Henry Morely. London: George Routledge p. 94

[164] Lohantan. 1703. *New Voyages to North-America: Giving a full account of the Customs, Commerce, Religion and strange Opinions of the Savages of that Country*. Vol 2. London. Available from: http://www.archive.org/details/cihm_37430

[165] Obomsawin R. 1983. Traditional Life Styles and Freedom from The Dark Seas of Disease. *Community Dev J*. 18(2):187-97

[166] Cordain L, Miller JB, Eaton SB, Mann N, Holt SHA, Speth JD. 2000. Plant-animal subsistence ratios and macronutrient energy estimations in worldwide hunter-gatherer diets. *Am J Clin Nutr*. 71:682–92

[167] Jönsson T, Granfeldt Y, Ahrén B, Branell UC, Pålsson G, Hansson A, Söderström M, Lindeberg S. 2009. Beneficial effects of a Paleolithic diet on cardiovascular risk factors in type 2 diabetes: a randomized cross-over pilot study. *Cardiovasc Diabetol*. 8:35

[168] Singh RB, Dubnov G, Niaz MA, et al. 2002. Effect of an Indo-Mediterranean diet on progression of coronary artery disease in high risk patients (Indo-Mediterranean Diet Heart Study): a randomised single-blind trial. *Lancet*. 360:1455-1461

[169] Ibid.

[170] Bajracharya MB. 2003. *Eastern Theory of Diet*. 3rd ed. Kathmandu: Piyushavarshi Aushadhalaya

[171] Beezhold BL, Johnston CS, Daigle DR. 2010. Vegetarian diets are associated with healthy mood states: a cross-sectional study in seventh day adventist adults. *Nutr J.* 9:26

[172] Lindbloom EJ. 2009. Long-term benefits of a vegetarian diet. *Am Fam Physician.* 79(7):541-2

[173] Fraser GE. 2009. Vegetarian diets: what do we know of their effects on common chronic diseases? *Am J Clin Nutr.* 89(5):1607S-1612S

[174] Giem P, Beeson WL, Fraser GE. 1993. The incidence of dementia and intake of animal products: preliminary findings from the Adventist Health Study. *Neuroepidemiology.* 12(1):28-36

[175] Ginter E. 2008. Vegetarian diets, chronic diseases and longevity. *Bratisl Lek Listy.* 109(10):463-6

[176] Lea E, Worsley A. 2003. The factors associated with the belief that vegetarian provide health benefits. *Asia Pac J Clin Nutr.* 12(3):296-303

[177] Weaver CM. 2009. Should dairy be recommended as part of a healthy vegetarian diet? Point. *Am J Clin Nutr.* 89(5):1634S-1637S

[178] Tapsell LC, Hemphill I, Cobiac L, Patch CS, Sullivan DR, Fenech M, Roodenrys S, Keogh JB, Clifton PM, Williams PG, Fazio VA, Inge KE. 2006. Health benefits of herbs and spices: the past, the present, the future. *Med J Aust.* 185(4 Suppl):S4-24

[179] Kohler K. 1901-06. *"Essenes"* in The Jewish Encyclopedia. New York: Funk and Wagnalls

[180] Li D. 2011. Chemistry behind Vegetarianism. *J Agric Food Chem.* [Epub ahead of print]

[181] Craig WJ. 2009. Health effects of vegan diets. *Am J Clin Nutr.* 89(5):1627S-1633S.

[182] Hipkiss AR. 2006. Would carnosine or a carnivorous diet help suppress aging and associated pathologies? *Ann N Y Acad Sci.* 1067:369-74

[183] Billings T. 1999. "Failure to Thrive (FTT)", in *Beyond Vegetarianism: Transcending Outdated Dogmas.* Accessed 11 Jan 2001. Available from: http://www.beyondveg.com/billings-t/comp-anat/comp-anat-9b.shtml

[184] Koebnick C, Strassner C, Hoffmann I, Leitzmann C. 1999. Consequences of a Long-Term Raw Food Diet on Body Weight and Menstruation: Results of a Questionnaire Survey. *Annals of Nutrition & Metabolism.* 43:69-79

[185] Ambroszkiewicz J, Klemarczyk W, Gajewska J, Chelchowska M, Franek E, Laskowska-Klita T. 2010. The influence of vegan diet on bone mineral density and biochemical bone turnover markers. *Pediatr Endocrinol Diabetes Metab.* 16(3):201-204

[186] Krivosíková Z, Krajcovicová-Kudlácková M, Spustová V, Stefíková K, Valachovicová M, Blazícek P, N mcová T. 2010. The association between high plasma homocysteine levels and lower bone mineral density in Slovak women: the impact of vegetarian diet. *Eur J Nutr.* 49(3):147-53

[187] Appleby P, Roddam A, Allen N, Key T. 2007. Comparative fracture risk in vegetarians and nonvegetarians in EPIC-Oxford. *Eur J Clin Nutr.* 61(12):1400-6

[188] Laffranchi L, Zotti F, Bonetti S, Dalessandri D, Fontana P. 2010. Oral implications of the vegan diet: observational study. *Minerva Stomatol.* 59(11-12):583-91

[189] Labay y Matías MV, Matamoros Florí N, Aguiló Regla A, Tomás Cardús L, Galiana Ferré C, Gómez Rivas B, Reynes Muntaner J. 1984. Strict vegetarian diet, malnutrition, immunodeficiency and infection. *An Esp Pediatr.* 20(1):69-71

[190] Baatenburg de Jong R, Bekhof J, Roorda R, Zwart P. 2005. Severe nutritional vitamin deficiency in a breast-fed infant of a vegan mother. *Eur J Pediatr.* 164(4):259-60

[191] Mariani A, Chalies S, Jeziorski E, Ludwig C, Lalande M, Rodière M. 2009. Consequences of exclusive breast-feeding in vegan mother newborn: case report *Arch Pediatr.* 16(11):1461-3

[192] Ferdowsian HR, Barnard ND, Hoover VJ, Katcher HI, Levin SM, Green AA, Cohen JL. 2010. A multicomponent intervention reduces body weight and cardiovascular risk at a GEICO corporate site. *Am J Health Promot.* 24(6):384-7

[193] Barnard ND, Cohen J, Jenkins DJ, Turner-McGrievy G, Gloede L, Green A, Ferdowsian H. 2009. A low-fat vegan diet and a conventional diabetes diet in the treatment of type 2 diabetes: a randomized, controlled, 74-wk clinical trial. *Am J Clin Nutr.* 89(5):1588S-1596S

[194] Barnard ND, Scialli AR, Turner-McGrievy G, Lanou AJ, Glass J. 2005. The effects of a low-fat, plant-based dietary intervention on body weight, metabolism, and insulin sensitivity. *Am J Med.* 118(9):991-7

[195] Jönsson T, Granfeldt Y, Erlanson-Albertsson C, Ahrén B, Lindeberg S. 2010. A paleolithic diet is more satiating per calorie than a mediterranean-like diet in individuals with ischemic heart disease. *Nutr Metab (Lond).* 30;7:85

[196] Jönsson T, Granfeldt Y, Ahrén B, Branell UC, Pålsson G, Hansson A, Söderström M, Lindeberg S. 2009. Beneficial effects of a Paleolithic diet on cardiovascular risk factors in type 2 diabetes: a randomized cross-over pilot study. *Cardiovasc Diabetol.* 8:35

[197] Klonoff DC. 2009. The beneficial effects of a Paleolithic diet on type 2 diabetes and other risk factors for cardiovascular disease. *J Diabetes Sci Technol.* 3(6): 1229-32

[198] Gardner CD, Kiazand A, Alhassan S, Kim S, Stafford RS, Balise RR, Kraemer HC, King AC. 2007. Comparison of the Atkins, Zone, Ornish, and LEARN diets for change in weight and related risk factors among overweight premenopausal women: the A TO Z Weight Loss Study: a randomized trial. *JAMA.* 297(9):969-77

[199] Arguin H, Sánchez M, Bray GA, Lovejoy JC, Peters JC, Jandacek RJ, Chaput JP, Tremblay A. 2010. Impact of adopting a vegan diet or an olestra supplementation on plasma organochlorine concentrations: results from two pilot studies. *Br J Nutr.* 103(10):1433-41

[200] Stefansson V. 1913. *My life with the Eskimo.* New York: MacMillan p. 176-8. Available online: http://openlibrary.org/books/OL6562100M/My_life_with_the_Eskimo

[201] Wrangham R, Conklin-Brittain N. 2003. Cooking as a biological trait. *Comp Biochem Physiol A Mol Integr Physiol.* 136(1):35-46.

[202] Carmody RN, Wrangham RW. 2009. The energetic significance of cooking. *J Hum Evol.* 57(4):379-91

[203] Mead PS, Slutsker L, Dietz V, McCaig LF, Bresee JS, Shapiro C, Griffin PM, Tauxe RV. 1999. Food-related illness and death in the United States. *Emerg Infect Dis.* 5(5):607-25

[204] Boback SM, Cox CL, Ott BD, Carmody R, Wrangham RW, Secor SM. 2007. Cooking and grinding reduces the cost of meat digestion. *Comp Biochem Physiol A Mol Integr Physiol.* 148(3):651-6

[205] Kumar R, Srivastava PK, Srivastava SP. 1994. Leaching of heavy metals (Cr, Fe, and Ni) from stainless steel utensils in food simulants and food materials. *Bull Environ Contam Toxicol.* 53(2):259-66

[206] Flint GN, Packirisamy S. 1997. Purity of food cooked in stainless steel utensils. *Food Addit Contam.* 14(2):115-26

[207] Kumar V, Gill KD. 2009. Aluminium neurotoxicity: neurobehavioural and oxidative aspects. *Arch Toxicol.* 83(11): 965-78

[208] Negri S, Maestri L, Esabon G, Ferrari M, Zadra P, Ghittori S, Imbriani M. 2008. Characteristics, use and toxicity of fluorochemicals: review of the literature. [Article in Italian] *G Ital Med Lav Ergon.* 30(1):61-74

[209] Frisbee SJ, Shankar A, Knox SS, Steenland K, Savitz DA, Fletcher T, Ducatman AM. 2010. Perfluorooctanoic acid, perfluorooctanesulfonate, and serum lipids in children and adolescents: results from the C8 Health Project. *Arch Pediatr Adolesc Med.* 164(9):860-9

[210] Doering C. "U.S. Urged to Put Warning Labels on Teflon Pans," Reuters 14 March 2003. Available from: http://www.ewg.org/news/us-urged-put-warning-labels-teflon-pans

[211] Toyama K, Kimura K, Miyashita M, Yanagisawa R, Nakata K. 2006. Case of lung edema occurring as a result of inhalation of fumes from a Teflon-coated flying pan overheated for 4 hours [Article in Japanese]. *Nihon Kokyuki Gakkai Zasshi.* 44(10):727-31

[212] "KRYTOX" LVP Fluorinated Grease, MSDS Number DU002667. Available from http://www.duniway.com/images/pdf/pg/MSDS-KRYTOX-Grease.pdf

[213] Goulas AE, Zygoura P, Karatapanis A, Georgantelis D, Kontominas MG. 2007. Migration of di(2-ethylhexyl) adipate and acetyltributyl citrate plasticizers from food-grade PVC film into sweetened sesame paste (halawa tehineh): kinetic and penetration study. *Food Chem Toxicol.* 45(4):585-91

[214] Cao XL, Corriveau J, Popovic S. 2010. Bisphenol a in canned food products from canadian markets. *J Food Prot.* 73(6):1085-9.

[215] Petersen JH, Jensen LK. 2008. Phthalates and food-contact materials: enforcing the 2008 European Union plastics legislation. *Food Addit Contam Part A Chem Anal Control Expo Risk Assess.* 27(11):1608-16.

[216] Vogel SA. 2009. The politics of plastics: the making and unmaking of bisphenol a "safety". *Am J Public Health.* 99 Suppl 3:S559-66.

[217] Crinnion WJ. 2010. Toxic effects of the easily avoidable phthalates and parabens. *Altern Med Rev.* 15(3):190-6.

[218] Ghisari M, Bonefeld-Jorgensen EC. 2009. Effects of plasticizers and their mixtures on estrogen receptor and thyroid hormone functions. *Toxicol Lett.* 189(1):67-77.

[219] López-Carrillo L, Hernández-Ramírez RU, Calafat AM, Torres-Sánchez L, Galván-Portillo M, Needham LL, Ruiz-Ramos R, Cebrián ME. 2010. Exposure to

phthalates and breast cancer risk in northern Mexico. *Environ Health Perspect.* 118(4):539-44.

[220] Prins GS, Tang WY, Belmonte J, Ho SM. 2008. Perinatal exposure to oestradiol and bisphenol A alters the prostate epigenome and increases susceptibility to carcinogenesis. *Basic Clin Pharmacol Toxicol.* 102(2):134-8.

[221] Grün F. 2010. Obesogens. *Curr Opin Endocrinol Diabetes Obes.* 17(5):453-9.

[222] Bornehag CG, Nanberg E. 2010. Phthalate exposure and asthma in children. *Int J Androl.* 33(2):333-45

[223] Hajszan T, Leranth C. 2010. Bisphenol A interferes with synaptic remodeling. *Front Neuroendocrinol.* 31(4):519-30.

[224] Martino-Andrade AJ, Chahoud I. 2010. Reproductive toxicity of phthalate esters. *Mol Nutr Food Res.* 54(1):148-57.

[225] Weuve J, Hauser R, Calafat AM, Missmer SA, Wise LA. 2010. Association of exposure to phthalates with endometriosis and uterine leiomyomata: findings from NHANES, 1999-2004. *Environ Health Perspect.* 118(6):825-32.

[226] Wagner M, Oehlmann J. 2009. Endocrine disruptors in bottled mineral water: total estrogenic burden and migration from plastic bottles. *Environ Sci Pollut Res Int.* 16(3):278-86

[227] Burros M. "Hot Stuff", New York Times 10 Jan 2007. Available from: www.nytimes.com/2007/01/10/dining/10sili.html

[228] USFDA Food Code 3-402.11

[229] Walker AR, Arvidsson UB. 1951. A comparison of the vitamin C content of vegetable stew when prepared on a large scale in open and pressure cookers. *Br J Nutr.* 5(2):167-70

[230] Chappell GM, Hamilton AM. 1949. Effect of pressure cooking on vitamin C content of vegetables. *Br Med J.* 1(4604):574

[231] Ramasamy R, Vannucci SJ, Yan SS, Herold K, Yan SF, Schmidt AM. 2005. Advanced glycation end products and RAGE: a common thread in aging, diabetes, neurodegeneration, and inflammation. *Glycobiology.* 15(7):16R-28R

[232] Peppa M, Uribarri J, Vlassara H. 2003. Glucose, Advanced Glycation End Products, and Diabetes Complications: What Is New and What Works. *Clinical Diabetes* 21:186-187

[233] Exon JH. 2006. A review of the toxicology of acrylamide. *J Toxicol Environ Health B Crit Rev.* 9(5):397-412

[234] Guillén MD, Goicoechea E. 2008. Toxic oxygenated alpha,beta-unsaturated aldehydes and their study in foods: a review. *Crit Rev Food Sci Nutr.* 48(2):119-36

[235] Zheng W, Lee SA. 2009. Well-done meat intake, heterocyclic amine exposure, and cancer risk. *Nutr Cancer.* 61(4):437-46

[236] Kozłowski J. 1993. Gas cookers as a source of benz(a)pyrene emission. *Rocz Panstw Zakl Hig.* 44(2-3):277-9

[237] Kabir E, Kim KH, Ahn JW, Hong OF, Sohn JR. 2010. Barbecue charcoal combustion as a potential source of aromatic volatile organic compounds and carbonyls. *J Hazard Mater.* 174(1-3):492-9

[238] Susaya J, Kim KH, Ahn JW, Jung MC, Kang CH. 2010. BBQ charcoal combustion as an important source of trace metal exposure to humans. *J Hazard Mater.* 176(1-3):932-7

[239] Pandey SK, Kim KH, Kang CH, Jung MC, Yoon H. 2008. BBQ charcoal as an important source of mercury emission. *J Hazard Mater.* 2009 Feb 15;162(1):536-8

[240] Salmon CP, Knize MG, Felton JS. Effects of marinating on heterocyclic amine carcinogen formation in grilled chicken. *Food Chem Toxicol.* 35.5 (1997): 433-441

[241] Shin IS, Rodgers WJ, Gomaa EA, Strasburg GM, Gray JI. Inhibition of heterocyclic aromatic amine formation in fried ground beef patties by garlic and selected garlic-related sulfur compounds. *J Food Prot.* 65.11 (2002): 1766-1770

[242] Forsythe P, Bienenstock J. 2010. Immunomodulation by commensal and probiotic bacteria. *Immunol Invest.* 39(4-5):429-48.

[243] Musso G, Gambino R, Cassader M. 2010. Obesity, diabetes, and gut microbiota: the hygiene hypothesis expanded? *Diabetes Care.* 33(10):2277-84.

[244] Lionetti E, Indrio F, Pavone L, Borrelli G, Cavallo L, Francavilla R. 2010. Role of probiotics in pediatric patients with *Helicobacter pylori* infection: a comprehensive review of the literature. *Helicobacter.* 15(2):79-87.

[245] Romeo MG, Romeo DM, Trovato L, Oliveri S, Palermo F, Cota F, Betta P. 2011. Role of probiotics in the prevention of the enteric colonization by Candida in preterm newborns: incidence of late-onset sepsis and neurological outcome. *J Perinatol.* 31(1):63-9.

[246] Liang J, Han BZ, Nout MJR, Hamer RJ. 2008. Effects of soaking, germination and fermentation on phytic acid, total and in vitro soluble zinc in brown rice. *Food Chemistry.* 110(4): 821-828

[247] Sharma A, Sehgal s. 1992. Effect of processing and cooking on the antinutritional factors of faba bean (Vicia faba). *Food Chemistry.* 43(5):383-385

[248] FAO. 1990. Manual on simple methods of meat preservation. Available from: http://www.fao.org/docrep/003/x6932e/x6932e00.htm

[249] USDA. 2006. Jerky and Food Safety. Available from: http://www.fsis.usda.gov/factsheets/jerky_and_food_safety/index.asp

[250] Duedahl-Olesen L, Christensen JH, Højgård A, Granby K, Timm-Heinrich M. 2010. Influence of smoking parameters on the concentration of polycyclic aromatic hydrocarbons (PAHs) in Danish smoked fish. *Food Addit Contam Part A Chem Anal Control Expo Risk Assess.* 27(9):1294-305.

[251] He FJ, MacGregor GA. 2009. A comprehensive review on salt and health and current experience of worldwide salt reduction programmes. *J Hum Hypertens.* 23(6):363-84.

[252] Tsugane S. 2005. Salt, salted food intake, and risk of gastric cancer: epidemiologic evidence. *Cancer Sci.* 96(1):1-6.

[253] de la Monte SM, Neusner A, Chu J, Lawton M. 2009. Epidemilogical trends strongly suggest exposures as etiologic agents in the pathogenesis of sporadic Alzheimer's disease, diabetes mellitus, and non-alcoholic steatohepatitis. *J Alzheimers Dis.* 17(3):519-29.

[254] Xie TP, Zhao YF, Chen LQ, Zhu ZJ, Hu Y, Yuan Y. 2011. Long-term exposure to sodium nitrite and risk of esophageal carcinoma: a cohort study for 30 years. *Dis Esophagus.* 24(1):30-2

[255] Hobbs C. 1995. *Medicinal Mushrooms: An Exploration of Tradition, Healing and Culture.* Loveland: Interweave Press. p 125-138

[256] Wettasinghe M, Bolling B, Plhak L, Xiao H, Parkin K. 2002. Phase II enzyme-inducing and antioxidant activities of beetroot (Beta vulgaris L.) extracts from phenotypes of different pigmentation. *J Agric Food Chem.* 50(23):6704-9.

[257] Nyirády P, Sárdi E, Beko G, Szucs M, Horváth A, Székely E, Szentmihályi K, Romics I, Blázovics A. 2010. Effects of bioactive molecules of *Beta vulgaris* L. *ssp. esculenta* var. *rubra* on metastatic prostate cancer. *Orv Hetil.* 151(37):1495-503.

[258] Webb AJ, Patel N, Loukogeorgakis S, Okorie M, Aboud Z, Misra S, Rashid R, Miall P, Deanfield J, Benjamin N, MacAllister R, Hobbs AJ, Ahluwalia A. 2008. Acute blood pressure lowering, vasoprotective, and antiplatelet properties of dietary nitrate via bioconversion to nitrite. *Hypertension.* 51(3):784-90.

[259] Mitchell SC. 2001. Food idiosyncrasies: beetroot and asparagus. *Drug Metab Dispos.* 29(4 Pt 2):539-43

[260] Ghosh S, Sanyal SN. 1956. Further clinical results with m-xylohydroquinone as an oral contraceptive. *Acta Endocrinol Suppl (Copenh).* 23(Suppl 28):83-92

[261] Personal communication. Heather Nic An Fhleisdeir, Medical Herbalist. 16 Jan 2011

[262] Cheney G, 1949. Rapid healing of peptic ulcers in patients receiving fresh cabbage juice. *California Medicine* 70 (10).

[263] Cheung KL, Kong AN. 2010. Molecular targets of dietary phenethyl isothiocyanate and sulforaphane for cancer chemoprevention. *AAPS J.* 12(1):87-97.

[264] Costello MJ. 2009. How sea lice from salmon farms may cause wild salmonid declines in Europe and North America and be a threat to fishes elsewhere. *Proc Biol Sci.* 276(1672):3385-94.

[265] Navarrete P, Mardones P, Opazo R, Espejo R, Romero J. 2008. Oxytetracycline treatment reduces bacterial diversity of intestinal microbiota of Atlantic salmon. *J Aquat Anim Health 20(3):177-83.*

[266] Kelly BC, Ikonomou MG, Higgs DA, Oakes J, Dubetz C. 2008. Mercury and other trace elements in farmed and wild salmon from British Columbia, Canada. *Environ Toxicol Chem.* 27(6):1361-70.

[267] Carlson DL, Hites RA. 2005. Polychlorinated biphenyls in salmon and salmon feed: global differences and bioaccumulation. *Environ Sci Technol.* 39(19):7389-95.

[268] http://www.cbc.ca/thelens/bigfatdiet/wortman.html

[269] Wagner M, Oehlmann J. 2009. Endocrine disruptors in bottled mineral water: total estrogenic burden and migration from plastic bottles. *Environ Sci Pollut Res.* 16(3):278-86

[270] Jamnicki T, Jamnicki S. 2011. Migration of itx (Isopropyl Thioxantone) from Tetra Pak Bricks into Food. *Acta Graphica.* 21(1-2):7-13

[271] Bailey DG, Malcolm J, Arnold O, Spence JD. 1998. Grapefruit juice-drug interactions. *Br J Clin Pharmacol.* 46(2):101-10

[272] Mannel M. 2004. Drug interactions with St John's Wort : mechanisms and clinical implications. *Drug Saf.* 27(11):773-97

[273] Powell JJ, Faria N, Thomas-McKay E, Pele LC. 2010. Origin and fate of dietary nanoparticles and microparticles in the gastrointestinal tract. *J Autoimmun.* 34(3):J226-33.

[274] Derikx JP, Luyer MD, Heineman E, Buurman WA. 2010. Non-invasive markers of gut wall integrity in health and disease. *World J Gastroenterol.* 16(42):5272-9.

[275] Soeters PB, Luyer MD, Greve JW, Buurman WA. 2007. The significance of bowel permeability. *Curr Opin Clin Nutr Metab Care.* 10(5):632-8.

[276] De Keyser F, Baeten D, Van Den Bosch F, De Vos M, Cuvelier C, Mielants H, Veys E. 2002. Gut inflammation and spondyloarthropathies. *Curr Rheumatol Rep.* 4(6):525-32

[277] Burns JJ, Zhao L, Taylor EW, Spelman K. 2010. The influence of traditional herbal formulas on cytokine activity. *Toxicology.* 278(1):140-59.

[278] Miller, SB. 1998. IgG Food Allergy Testing by ELISA/EIA What Do They Really Tell Us? *Townsend Lett Doc Pat.* 174:62-65

Index

A

abdominal pain, 52
açaí, 217
acesulfame-k, 79
acid reflux, 31
acne, 62, 132, 136, 232
acrylamide, 120
Addison's disease, 52
adrenals, 129, 149
adzuki, 181
aflatoxins, 59
aging, 11, 19, 56, 105, 120, 129, 138, 139, 195, 214
agni, 14
agrarian revolution, 94
agrarianism, 50
ahimsa, 102
ajwain, 27, 141, 155, 181, 182, 187, 198
alcohol, 68, 84, 85, 86, 87, 88, 129, 202, 215, 220
alfalfa sprouts, 41
allergy, 59, 97
almond milk, 191
almond oil, 75
alpha-lactalbumin, 62
alteratives, 224
Alzheimer's disease, 128
ama, 15, 28, 38, 61, 64, 65, 66, 75, 106, 150, 176, 222
amaranth greens, 41, 153, 155
amchur (unripe mango powder), 198
American ginseng, 129, 149, 165, 166, 199, 200, 235, 237, 241, 242, 243, 245
amla, 44, 86, 129, 232, 233, 234, 235, 236, 237, 238, 239, 240, 242, 244, 245, 246
anardana (pomegranate seed powder), 198
anemia, 38, 52, 79, 106, 138, 139, 151, 174, 199, 232
angelica, 132
anise, 202
Ann Wigmore, 106
annatto, 168
antinutrient factors (ANFs), 50, 59, 121, 126, 191
antioxidant, 42, 78, 82, 128, 162, 183, 278
anxiety, 21, 52, 53, 130, 139

aperients, 224
apéritifs, 202
aphrodisiacs, 86, 130, 132, 135, 137, 138, 181, 201, 203
appetite, 25, 28, 42, 66, 79, 83, 130, 132, 134, 135, 140, 161, 202, 212, 218, 223
arachidonic acid (AA), 71
arame, 154
arishta, 87
arjun, 174
arrhythmia, 56
arterial disease, 239
arthritis, 52, 62, 71, 84, 97, 104, 136, 137, 147, 173, 174, 218, 233, 274
artichoke, 41
asafoetida, 130
asava, 88
Ashtanga Hrdaya, 84
ashwagandha, 130, 174, 201, 202, 232, 235, 236, 237, 238, 240, 241, 242, 243, 244, 245, 246
Asian kitchari, 181
asparagus, 41
aspartame, 79
asthma, 27, 38, 71, 78, 113, 130, 137, 138, 174, 233, 284
astragalus, 55, 130, 149, 165, 166, 199, 200, 203, 234, 236, 239, 241, 242, 243, 244, 245
astringent, 24, 25
Atreya, 11
atta, 186
autoimmunity, 52, 97
autumn, 27
Ayurveda, 13
    and diet, 98

B

bacterial infection, 197
bai he, 137
bala, 174
bananas, 30
barberry, 75, 86, 224, 226
basil, 29, 41, 42, 43, 101, 121, 130, 143, 156, 160, 168, 169, 188, 197, 217, 218, 237, 244
basmati rice, 183
bay, 41, 131, 143, 152, 168, 169, 181, 182, 239, 244

bay leaves, 41, 131, 152, 168, 169, 181, 182
bayberry, 223
beef, 30
beet greens, 41, 154, 217
beet root, 41, 151
beeturia, 151
bell pepper, 41, 42, 160
beta-lactoglobulin, 62
bibhitaki, 87, 225, 226
biotin, 30
bison, 165
bitter, 24, 25
bitter melon, 217, 218, 236, 238
black cumin, 134
black mustard, 43, 131, 149, 150, 154, 155, 162, 170, 178, 181, 182, 187, 244
black pepper, 118, 131, 149, 153, 155, 157, 159, 164, 165, 166, 167, 168, 169, 170, 171, 172, 173, 175, 178, 180, 181, 187, 198, 201, 202, 223, 244
black rice, 183
bladder infection, 134
bladderwrack, 41, 140
bleeding, 66, 133, 139
bloating, 31, 38, 57, 62, 79, 130, 131, 134, 135, 138, 141, 159, 172, 202, 223
blood, 25, 29, 31, 37, 40, 42, 43, 46, 47, 50, 66, 68, 74, 130, 132, 133, 135, 136, 137, 138, 139, 141, 151, 171, 184, 199, 209, 214, 216, 218, 224
Blood Building Syrup, 199
blood sugar, 29, 40, 46, 50, 98, 132, 133, 135, 141, 216
blurred vision, 139
Boiled Milk, 173
bok choy, 41, 118, 153, 154
bone density, 106
bone fracture, 106
Borscht, 151
bowel, 211, 218, 222
bowel movement, 32
brain damage, 36
breakfast, 29
Breakfast Bowl, 151, 182
breast milk
    and pollutants, 47
breastfeeding, 48, 134, 141
breastmilk, 135
broccoli, 41, 42, 117, 149, 156, 182, 218
broccoli sprouts, 41
bronchitis, 78, 173, 174

Brown Basmati Pullao, 183
bruises, 78
brussel sprout, 41
bu gu zhi, 55
Buddhism, 102
buplerum, 224
burdock, 41, 224
burdock root, 232, 240
Burgundy Bitters, 202
burning sensations, 27, 42, 61, 66, 79, 174
burping, 31
buttermilk, 27, 65, 100, 176, 177, 178
butternut squash, 156

C

cabbage, 41, 101, 118, 151, 152, 154, 159, 161, 164, 217, 218, 286
caffeine, 80, 82, 83, 84
calcium, 62
calendula, 131, 232, 234, 236, 239, 242, 243, 246
calories, 11
cancer, 11, 36, 40, 46, 50, 52, 55, 56, 59, 62, 64, 68, 71, 73, 77, 79, 80, 96, 113, 122, 124, 128, 151, 274, 275, 278
candidiasis, 88, 98
caraway, 131, 143, 152, 159, 234, 236, 237, 238
carbohydrates, 30
cardamom, 65, 131, 132, 143, 157, 158, 170, 173, 180, 183, 184, 191, 196, 199, 200, 201, 202, 203, 204, 223, 236, 237, 239, 241, 242, 244
cardiovascular disease, 46, 50, 62, 64, 68, 71, 73, 77, 80, 96, 98, 113, 120, 122, 128, 151, 167, 174, 218, 272, 277, 282
carob, 236
carrot pickle, 161
cascara sagrada, 225, 226
casein protein, 63
cauliflower, 41, 187
cayenne, 27, 38, 132, 151, 158, 168, 198, 223, 233, 234, 235, 237, 239, 241, 242, 244, 246
celery, 27, 30, 41, 118, 119, 132, 150, 152, 168, 169, 170, 171, 217
celiac disease, 52
cereal grains, 49
chai, 173
chamomile, 203
Charaka samhita, 11
chard, 24, 41, 118, 154, 155, 217, 218

cheese, 30
chemotherapy, 199
chen pi, 138
chestnuts, 30
chickweed, 132, 232, 234, 236, 238, 239, 243, 246
childhood, 19, 74
children, 106
chili, 24, 101, 132, 155, 162, 163, 164, 165, 168, 187, 197
Chinese ginseng, 132, 203
Chinese red date, 232, 245
Chinese red dates, 133
Chinese yam, 133, 234, 242, 243
chipotle, 164, 168, 169
chocolate, 82, 83, 201, 202, 279
cholagogues, 223, 226
choy sum, 153
cilantro, 41, 118, 133, 150, 151, 155, 163, 164, 166, 169, 171, 172, 175, 181, 182, 186, 199, 217, 218
cinnamon, 65, 133, 143, 157, 158, 165, 166, 167, 168, 170, 173, 180, 183, 184, 188, 192, 196, 199, 200, 201, 202, 203, 204, 223, 233, 236, 239, 241, 242, 245
circulation, 17, 38, 131, 132, 133, 135, 136, 137, 138, 139, 140, 141, 161, 165, 168, 218, 223
cirrhosis, 85
cleavers, 224
Clostridium, 125
clove, 133, 157, 158, 165, 166, 168, 170, 173, 183, 184, 196, 199, 200, 201, 202, 203, 204
coconut chutney, 190
coconut oil, 75
coconut smoothie, 192
codonopsis, 133, 234, 239, 241, 242
coffee, 83
    espresso, 83
coffee substitute, 134
cold sores, 66
coldness, 132
colds, 27, 38, 131, 135, 137, 140, 141, 149, 174, 203, 234
cold-smoking, 128
colic, 131, 132, 133, 134, 135, 137, 141, 218
complexion, 194
congee, 180
constipation, 17, 32, 37, 38, 40, 50, 52, 55, 61, 62, 125, 134, 135, 136, 140, 234
constitution, 16

convulsions, 38
cookware, 109
    and aluminum, 112
    and cast iron, 111
    and ceramics, 109
    and copper, 111
    and glass, 112
    and plastic, 113
    and polytetrafluoroethylene (Teflon), 113
    and silicone, 114
    and soapstone, 110
    and stainless steel, 112
coriander, 133, 143, 149, 150, 155, 158, 159, 162, 170, 172, 175, 181, 182, 187, 189, 198, 202, 236, 237, 238, 240, 242
couch grass, 225
cough, 27, 38, 66, 78, 129, 130, 132, 134, 135, 136, 137, 138, 140, 141, 173, 197, 234
cow's milk, 65
crab, 30
cranberries, 185
cream, 176
creamery butter, 176
crème fraiche, 157
Crohn's disease, 97
cucumber, 30, 41, 162, 175, 182, 217
Cucurbitaceae, 156
Cultured Butter, 176
cumin, 43, 134, 143, 149, 150, 154, 155, 157, 158, 162, 167, 168, 169, 170, 171, 175, 178, 180, 181, 182, 183, 184, 187, 189, 190, 198, 237, 244
curing, 127
curry, 170
curry leaf, 41, 134, 155, 170, 178

D

daidzein
    and soy, 56
daikon, 24, 40, 41, 101, 162, 163, 165, 166
dairy, 61
damiana, 203
dandelion, 41, 134, 225, 226
dandelion root, 232, 240, 246
dang gui, 132, 148, 171, 203, 232, 242, 243, 244, 245
deficiency, 165, 189, 191, 195, 197, 215, 216
dementia, 51, 52, 56, 82, 104, 136, 234, 279

dental problems, 106
deodorization, 72
depression, 82, 235, 273, 274
dermatitis herpetiformis, 52
detoxification, 15, 31, 58, 106, 108, 115,
    133, 140, 148, 150, 151, 153, 180,
    209, 210, 211, 213, 214, 220, 222,
    223, 225, 226
Dhaniya Chicken, 172
diabetes, 39, 46, 50, 52, 54, 62, 64, 68,
    73, 74, 77, 81, 82, 94, 96, 98, 104,
    105, 106, 120, 122, 128, 129, 137,
    167, 218, 219, 235, 271, 273, 277,
    280, 282
    and cereal grains, 50
diaphoretics, 225
diarrhea, 27, 32, 51, 56, 61, 62, 66, 125,
    130, 133, 137, 174, 177, 236
digestifs, 202
digestion, 15, 16, 17, 20, 21, 25, 26, 30,
    31, 32, 37, 42, 43, 46, 50, 52, 54, 57,
    58, 61, 65, 66, 67, 74, 75, 78, 97, 104,
    107, 108, 115, 126, 130, 131, 133,
    134, 135, 136, 138, 139, 140, 141,
    147, 149, 150, 156, 162, 165, 168,
    177, 180, 181, 196, 202, 211, 212,
    216, 218, 219, 220, 225
dill, 27, 118, 134, 143, 159, 167, 171,
    184, 217, 223, 236, 237, 244
diuretics, 225
dizziness, 138, 140
docosahexaenoic acid (DHA), 71
doshas, 15
douchi, 56, 57, 154
dried fruit, 43
dryness, 195
dulse, 41, 140, 147, 149, 154
dyspnea, 132

E

earth, 13, 24
eczema, 62, 132, 136, 236
edema, 58, 113, 134, 135, 139, 149
Edward Howell, 106
eggplant, 41
eicosanoids, 71
eicosapentaenoic acid (EPA), 71
elecampane, 225, 226
electrolytes, 138, 140, 150, 153
elements, 24
elevated insulin, 46
elimination-challenge diet, 231
encephalization quotient
    and raw food, 107

epazoté, 134, 164, 168, 169
epigallocatechin gallate (EGCG), 80
epilepsy, 52, 130, 273
erythritol, 79
excess mucus, 27, 67, 74, 130, 131, 132,
    135, 138, 163, 173, 198, 225
exhaustion, 38, 74, 136, 140, 173, 174,
    199
expectorants, 225
eyes, 74, 184, 218

F

failure-to-thrive syndrome, 106
fasting, 213
fat, 67
fatigue, 38, 52, 79, 106, 129, 133, 135,
    140, 174, 212, 220
fats, 30
fatty acids, 68
fatty liver, 85
fennel, 135, 143, 155, 165, 167, 173,
    174, 203, 223, 234, 235, 236, 242
fenugreek, 41, 135, 143, 155, 170, 178,
    186, 196, 234, 236, 237, 239, 242,
    244
fermentation
    and cereal and legumes, 126
    and dairy, 126
    and sourdough, 127
    and vegetables, 126
fertility, 55, 58, 130, 135, 174
fever, 27, 38, 61, 66, 74, 129, 134, 135,
    136, 137, 139, 140, 177, 237
fibromyalgia, 52, 237
fiddlehead, 41
field mint, 137
fire, 13, 24
fish, 29, 30
fish oil, 75
fish sauce, 161
five-spice, 165
Five-spice Bison Stew, 165
flu, 27, 38, 135, 141, 149
food allergies, 151, 220, 231, 237
food combinations, 29
food preparation
    baking, 119
    boiling, 118
    braising, 118
    deep-frying, 123
    drying, 127
    fermentation, 125
    germination, 116
    grilling, 124

raw food, 115
roasting, 119
salting, 128
sautéing, 123
smoking, 128
steaming, 117
stewing, 118
stir-frying, 122
food quantity and timing, 28
food sensitivities, 231
fortified wines, 202
fringetree, 224
fruit, 43
fu ling, 139, 149
fungal infection, 197

G

gai lan, 41, 153, 156
gall bladder, 218
gall bladder problems, 32
gallstones, 134, 238
garlic, 27, 29, 40, 41, 42, 43, 101, 117,
    118, 124, 130, 131, 135, 143, 149,
    150, 151, 152, 154, 156, 158, 160,
    161, 163, 164, 165, 166, 167, 168,
    169, 170, 171, 174, 175, 178, 181,
    196, 197, 217, 224, 233, 234, 236,
    239, 243, 244, 246, 257, 285
Garlic Herb Oil, 196
garlic sprouts, 41
gastroenteritis, 125
genistein
    and soy, 56
gentian, 202
ghee, 29, 43, 61, 62, 72, 73, 74, 78, 86,
    96, 99, 100, 104, 122, 123, 131, 155,
    157, 158, 170, 171, 177, 178, 180,
    182, 184, 194, 195, 196, 199, 200,
    202, 220
ginger, 27, 40, 41, 42, 43, 65, 86, 101,
    118, 135, 143, 149, 151, 154, 155,
    156, 157, 158, 161, 162, 163, 165,
    166, 170, 171, 173, 181, 182, 196,
    202, 204, 217, 218, 223, 226, 233,
    234, 235, 236, 237, 238, 239, 241,
    242, 243, 244, 245, 246
ginseng, 235, 236
gluconeogenesis
    and meat, 46
glucosamine, 147
gluten, 51
gluten intolerance, 52
glycotoxins, 108, 120, 122, 123, 124
glycyrrhizin, 79

goat, 169
Goat Curry, 169
goat's milk, 66
gobi parantha, 187
goji, 135, 174, 184, 185, 199, 232, 235,
    240, 242, 243, 244, 245
Goji Quinoa Pilaf, 184
gokshura, 225
gomashio, 189
gotu kola, 235, 236, 240, 243
gout, 94, 132, 137, 238
Greek salad, 153
guacamole, 164
gum recession, 84

H

habañero, 168
hair, 149, 189, 191
hair loss, 56, 66
halal, 169
haldi, 141
half-sweet fruits, 44
hangover, 85
haritaki, 225
hay fever, 238
he shou wu, 138
headache, 37, 84, 135, 137, 173, 212,
    220
heart disease, 239
heartburn, 31, 239
heavy metals, 218
hemorrhage, 38, 129
hemorrhoids, 50, 66, 132, 135, 177, 240
hemp, 60, 61, 71, 73, 121, 122, 136,
    183, 192, 198, 234
hepatitis, 85, 108, 129, 136
Herbert Shelton, 106
Herring's Law, 221
heterocyclic amines, 108, 124
hiatus hernia, 31, 239
high blood sugar, 46
high cholesterol, 239
hijiki, 41, 140, 154
hin choy, 153, 155
hing, 130, 143, 155, 172, 178, 180, 181,
    182, 187, 189, 198, 233, 236, 237,
    244
holy basil, 136, 233, 234, 235, 236, 237,
    239, 244
homogenization, 63
honey, 29, 66, 75, 76, 78, 79, 86, 87,
    105, 160, 174, 201, 202, 203
hops, 87
hot drinks, 29

liver disease, 59
long pepper, 137
lotus, 41
low blood pressure, 37
lungs, 129, 130, 133, 135, 211, 222, 225
luo han, 79
lymph, 209

M

maca, 201, 202
mace, 203
malabsorption, 52, 151
Mana Bajra Bajracharya, 98
Mango Chat, 198
Manu Smriti, 102
maple syrup, 77
marinade, 143
marjoram, 41, 137, 150, 203
marrow fat, 75, 195
masala, 131, 142, 169, 173, 198
masto khiar, 175
maté, 84
meat, 29, 45
Medicinal Mushroom Broth, 148
memory, 136
menopause, 130, 132, 138, 139, 148,
    243
mercury
    and fish, 48
metabolic syndrome, 50, 77
metabolism, 17, 26, 29, 37, 40, 43, 46,
    140, 147, 149, 162, 218, 282
methi, 41, 135, 155, 158, 186
Mexican Chicken stew, 167
migraine, 52, 274
milk, 29, 61
milk allergies, 63
mind, 194, 218
mint, 41, 137, 143, 164, 171, 175, 199,
    237, 238, 239
miso, 30, 56, 181
molasses, 79, 165, 199
molds, 43
monounsaturated fats, 69
    and cooking, 122
morita, 168
mucolytics, 225
mucus, 25, 78, 79, 131, 132, 133, 135,
    136, 138, 139, 140, 162, 209, 212,
    216, 218, 221, 225
mullein, 225
multiple sclerosis, 74, 97
mung, 180
mung sprouts, 41

musta, 223
mustard, 30, 159, 217
mustard greens, 42, 154, 218
Muttar panir, 157
m-xylohydroquinone, 157
mycotoxins, 59, 60, 82

N

nasturtium, 41
natto, 56
nausea, 31, 42, 131, 132, 134, 135, 138,
    173, 174
nervous system, 194
nettle, 37, 41, 137, 143, 148, 149, 189,
    224, 232, 234, 236, 237, 238, 239,
    242, 243, 245, 246, 260
neurodegeneration, 62, 106, 120, 122
neurotoxicity, 56, 283
Niter Kibbeh, 196
nitrate/nitrite, 128
nitrosamines, 108, 128
non-protein amino acids (NPAAs), 51,
    55, 56
non-starchy vegetables, 40
non-vegetarian, 98, 99, 103
nori, 41
Northwest Wild Rice Infusion, 185
nutmeg, 137, 138, 143, 157, 168, 173,
    188, 192, 196, 201, 202, 203, 204,
    237, 242, 243
nuts, 58

O

oatstraw, 149
obesity, 39, 46, 50, 62, 79, 98, 106, 113,
    243
offal, 49
oil infusion, 196
ojas, 14
Old-fashioned Sauerkraut, 159
olive oil, 75
omega 3, 64, 71, 75, 136, 166
omega 6, 64, 71
onion, 18, 30, 40, 41, 42, 101, 117, 149,
    150, 153, 157, 158, 159, 161, 163,
    164, 166, 171, 178, 184
onion sprouts, 41
orange peel, 138, 203, 223, 234, 238,
    239, 241, 242
oregano, 41, 42, 43, 118, 121, 137, 138,
    143, 151, 153, 164, 167, 168, 169,
    188, 197, 233, 234, 237, 239

organ meats, 49
organic, 33
organochlorines, 106
osteoporosis, 52, 106, 147, 244

P

Paenibacillus
   and pasteurized milk, 63
pain, 20, 21, 38, 84, 132, 133, 135, 137,
   138, 139, 141, 173, 174
paleolithic diet
   and restricted foods, 97
paleolithic diet, 96
pancake mix, 127
panch karma, 180
pancreatitis, 52, 273
panir, 66, 67, 104, 157, 158, 178, 179
papaya leaf, 223
paprika, 132, 167
paralysis, 56
parasites, 108, 116, 130, 134, 135, 139,
   141, 168, 244
Parkinson's disease, 55
parsley, 138, 150, 153, 167, 171, 175,
   184, 217, 218, 225
parsnip, 41
Parvati's Delight, 201
pasilla, 168
pasteurization, 62
pea, 157
peanut, 30
pellagra, 51
peony, 86, 138, 148, 171, 232, 234, 242,
   243, 244, 245
peppermint, 137
peripheral neuropathy, 52
Persian Lamb Shanks, 171
persimmon, 30
phytate, 50, 60
phytoestrogens
   and legumes, 55
   and soy, 56
Pickled Pepper Paste, 160
pink salt, 24, 138, 140, 143, 155, 170,
   198, 199, 200, 236
pippali, 137, 199, 200, 236, 237, 239,
   241, 242, 244
pipsissewa, 225
pitta, 16, 172, 176, 191, 215
   and alcohol, 88
   and cereal grains, 54
   and coffee, 83
   and fasting, 221
   and fruit, 45

and legumes, 58
and meat, 49
and nuts and seeds, 61
and vegetables, 42
and wine, 87
reducing diet, 100
pitta disease symptoms, 21
PMS, 134
Poaceae, 49
Poached Herb Wild Salmon, 166
poke root, 224
pollutants
   and meat, 47
polycyclic aromatic hydrocarbons
   (PAHs), 128
polygonum, 138
polymer fume fever', 113
polyphenols, 50
polyunsaturated fats, 69
   and cooking, 122
   and nuts and seeds, 58
poor fat digestion, 32
poor gastric motility, 31
poppy, 203
poria, 139, 244
pork, 30
post-partum, 173
post-partum exhaustion, 244
post-prandial dip, 29
prakriti, 16
   questionnaire, 255
prana, 14
pre-eclampsia, 82
pregnancy, 74, 106, 134, 141, 195
premenstrual syndrome, 104, 106, 134,
   138, 139, 157, 245
pressure cooker, 59, 119, 166, 169, 170,
   172, 182
prickly ash, 139
probiotic, 160, 161, 164, 176
prostatitis, 245
protease inhibitors, 50, 60
protein putrefaction, 31
proteins, 30
psoriasis, 52, 55, 273
punarnava, 86, 87
pungent, 24, 25

Q

quality, 14
quinoa, 55, 184, 200

R

rabbit, 30
radicchio, 41
radish, 29, 41
rapini, 41, 154, 156
raw foodism, 106, 107
raw fruit, 43
raw milk, 64, 176
red clover, 224, 226
red clover sprouts, 41
red meat, 46
red rice, 183
rehmannia, 139, 148, 199, 200, 232, 240, 243, 245, 246
rheumatism, 136
rhubarb, 41
rhubarb root, 225
rice sprouts, 223
Rig Veda, 102
rose, 81, 139, 175, 201, 235, 245
rosemary, 41, 118, 121, 139, 143, 160, 164, 188, 197, 233, 235, 239, 258
roti (chapatti), 186
rub, 143
rum, 204
rutabaga, 40, 41, 162, 219

S

saffron, 184
sage, 139
salivation, 25, 139
salmon, 166
Salsa, 164
salty, 24, 25
Samkhya darshana, 13
san choy, 153
sanchal, 138
Satmya, 65
saturated fats, 69
    and cooking, 122
savory, 126, 150, 159, 217
sea salt, 140
seaweed, 140, 147
seeds, 58
senna, 55, 225
serrano, 168
sesame oil, 75
shallot, 41
shan zha, 223
shatavari, 86, 130, 148, 149, 174, 199, 200, 201, 202, 234, 238, 242, 243, 244, 245

sheep's milk, 66
shiitake mushroom, 148, 165
shiso, 181
short-chain fatty acids, 30
shu, 139
sickle cell anemia, 232
sinus congestion, 62
skin, 74, 149, 189, 191, 194, 211, 222
skin disease, 136, 137
slippery elm, 140, 234, 239, 242, 246
Solomon's seal, 140, 234, 245
sore throat, 137, 141
soup stock, 147, 149
sour, 24, 25, 29
sourdough, 53, 127
soy, 56
space, 13, 24
spasm, 17, 21, 138, 173
spearmint, 137
Spicy Daikon Relish, 162
Spicy Saag, 154
spinach, 41, 118, 153, 154
spleen, 139
spring, 27
squash, 24, 41, 42, 60, 118, 120, 156, 157
star anise, 165, 166
starchy vegetables, 40
steatorrhea, 52
stevia, 79
stress, 16, 31, 84, 136, 174, 210, 211, 213, 219, 277, 278
substance abuse, 85
sucralose, 79
sui choy, 41, 153, 159
summer, 27
surgery, 199
suribachi, 189
sweating, 130, 140
sweet, 24, 25
sweet potato, 40, 41, 42, 97, 118
sweeteners, 76
Szechuan pepper, 139, 143, 165, 232, 237, 241

T

tahini, 157, 183, 201, 202
tallow, 75, 195
tamari, 43, 57, 100, 118, 126, 151, 154, 156, 157, 161, 165, 166, 181, 183
tamarind, 140, 232
taro, 30
tarragon, 141
tatziki, 175

tea, 79
  bancha, 81
  green tea, 81
  oolong tea, 81
  pu-erh, 81, 82
  red tea, 81
  white tea, 81
tejaphal, 139
tempeh, 56
Thai basil, 155
theanine, 80
theobromine, 80, 82, 83, 84
theophylline, 80, 83
thepla, 186
thirst, 37, 38, 79, 140
throat irritation, 38, 65
thyme, 41, 141, 143, 150, 197, 233, 234, 237
thyroid, 140
thyroid dysfunction, 36
tiger lily, 41
toasted sesame oil, 161, 165
tofu, 30, 56
tomatillos, 164
tomato, 41, 42, 101, 164, 178
toxins, 28, 47, 58, 59, 61, 76, 78, 108, 109, 150, 210, 211, 212, 214, 218, 219, 222, 224
transfats, 73, 108
tridosha, 15
triglycerides, 68
trihalomethanes, 36
triphala, 75, 226
trivrit, 225
true fir, 226
tulsi, 136, 225
turmeric, 40, 86, 141, 143, 149, 150, 155, 158, 170, 173, 175, 178, 180, 181, 182, 187, 196, 217, 218, 224, 232, 233, 234, 235, 236, 237, 238, 239, 240, 242, 244, 245, 246
turnip greens, 154

U

ulcers, 159, 174, 246
urad, 57, 58, 150, 181, 182
urinary problems, 132
uveitis, 52

V

varicose veins, 218

vata, 17, 165, 171, 176, 189, 191, 195, 215
  and alcohol, 88
  and cereal grains, 54
  and coffee, 83
  and fasting, 221
  and fruit, 45
  and legumes, 57
  and meat, 49
  and nuts and seeds, 61
  and vegetables, 43
  and wine, 87
  reducing diet, 99
vata disease symptoms, 21
vata-kapha, 18
vata-pitta, 18
vata-pitta-kapha, 18
veganism, 105
vegetables, 38
vegetarian, 46, 47, 98, 99, 101, 102, 103, 104, 157, 220, 272
vikriti, 19
vital deficiency, 74
vitality, 14, 15, 61, 74, 95, 103, 129, 130, 132, 133, 135, 138, 139
vitamin A toxicity, 49
vitamin B12, 30
vitamin D3, 48, 49
vitamin K2, 30

W

wakame, 41, 140
water, 13, 24, 34
  and toxins, 36
  artesian wells, 35
  chlorine, 36
  cold water, 38
  copper disinfection, 37
  distillation, 37
  fluoride, 36
  glacial water, 34
  rainwater, 34
  reverse osmosis membrane, 37
  solar water disinfection, 37
  surface water, 36
  warm water, 38
water buffalo milk, 66
water chestnut, 41
water fasting, 215
watercress, 41
weakness, 15, 20, 74, 79, 165, 173, 174
weaning, 66
weight loss, 37, 52, 74, 106, 140, 215
wheat allergies, 184

whiskey, 204
white sugar, 77
wild celery, 141
wild rice, 185
wind, 13, 24
wine, 86
winter, 26
winter melon, 217, 218, 260
winter squash, 156
withdrawal, 220
wormwood, 203
wounds, 132
wrinkled skin, 120

xylitol, 79

yarrow, 225
yeasts, 43
yogavahi, 75
yogurt, 66, 174, 179

CPSIA information can be obtained at www.ICGtesting.com
Printed in the USA
LVOW020540171112

307722LV00004B/2/P